PHACO MACHINE
and its Applications

DISCLOSURE

There is no financial interest in Phaco machine of any company.

PHACO MACHINE
and its Applications

Navneet Toshniwal
MBBS MS (Ophthalmology)
Director
Navneet Hospital
Solapur, Maharashtra, India

Foreword
Prof Keiki R Mehta

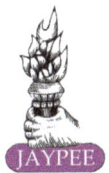

JAYPEE BROTHERS MEDICAL PUBLISHERS
The Health Sciences Publisher
New Delhi | London

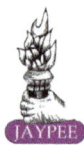 **Jaypee Brothers Medical Publishers (P) Ltd**

Headquarters

Jaypee Brothers Medical Publishers (P) Ltd
EMCA House, 23/23-B
Ansari Road, Daryaganj
New Delhi 110 002, India
Landline: +91-11-23272143, +91-11-23272703
+91-11-23282021, +91-11-23245672
Email: jaypee@jaypeebrothers.com

Corporate Office

Jaypee Brothers Medical Publishers (P) Ltd
4838/24, Ansari Road, Daryaganj
New Delhi 110 002, India
Phone: +91-11-43574357
Fax: +91-11-43574314
Email: jaypee@jaypeebrothers.com

Overseas Office

JP Medical Ltd
83 Victoria Street, London
SW1H 0HW (UK)
Phone: +44 20 3170 8910
Fax: +44 (0)20 3008 6180
Email: info@jpmedpub.com

Website: www.jaypeebrothers.com
Website: www.jaypeedigital.com

© 2022, Jaypee Brothers Medical Publishers

The views and opinions expressed in this book are solely those of the original contributor(s)/author(s) and do not necessarily represent those of editor(s) of the book.

All rights reserved. No part of this publication may be reproduced, stored or transmitted in any form or by any means, electronic, mechanical, photocopying, recording or otherwise, without the prior permission in writing of the publishers.

All brand names and product names used in this book are trade names, service marks, trademarks or registered trademarks of their respective owners. The publisher is not associated with any product or vendor mentioned in this book.

Medical knowledge and practice change constantly. This book is designed to provide accurate, authoritative information about the subject matter in question. However, readers are advised to check the most current information available on procedures included and check information from the manufacturer of each product to be administered, to verify the recommended dose, formula, method and duration of administration, adverse effects and contraindications. It is the responsibility of the practitioner to take all appropriate safety precautions. Neither the publisher nor the author(s)/editor(s) assume any liability for any injury and/or damage to persons or property arising from or related to use of material in this book.

This book is sold on the understanding that the publisher is not engaged in providing professional medical services. If such advice or services are required, the services of a competent medical professional should be sought.

Every effort has been made where necessary to contact holders of copyright to obtain permission to reproduce copyright material. If any have been inadvertently overlooked, the publisher will be pleased to make the necessary arrangements at the first opportunity. The **CD/DVD-ROM** (if any) provided in the sealed envelope with this book is complimentary and free of cost. **Not meant for sale.**

Inquiries for bulk sales may be solicited at: jaypee@jaypeebrothers.com

PHACO MACHINE **and its Applications**

First Edition: **2022**

ISBN: 978-93-5465-413-8

Dedicated to

*My dear wife
Mrs. Sunita Toshniwal*

Blessings

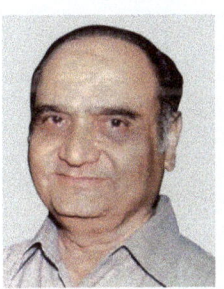

Late Dr Shamsundar Toshniwal
Founder
Navneet Hospital and Smt Misribai Gulabchand Toshniwal
Eye Bank Trust and Research Foundation
Solapur, Maharashtra, India

Foreword

I am indeed honored to be asked to write a foreword for Dr Navneet Toshniwal's fourth book on Phaco Machines. The fact that it is still in demand enough to write the fourth edition is proof of the necessity of this book.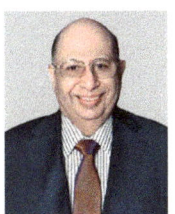

No other surgical specialty has been so dominated by a single surgical procedure as has phacoemulsification in cataract surgery. Cataract removal is a simple but extremely delicate procedure during which the intricate knowledge and capability of the phacoemulsification machines are so very essential. A single moment of inattention or an incorrect setting is likely to be catastrophic. Through a cooperative marriage of industrial engineering and the surgical innovation, the procedure has evolved exponentially, thanks to the inventive genius of Charles Kelman in 1967.

If one is to consider an analogy between Phacoemulsification and Formula 1 racing, the epitome of car racing in the world, the similarities are striking.

In both, intricate knowledge of the tools available are vitally important. In the case of the ophthalmologist, the nuances of the Phaco machine and how to achieve the maximum cause and effect combining his own skills complimented by the machine are important. For the Formula 1 driver, the knowledge of his car and its latent abilities are essential. Michael Schumacher, the seven-time world champion, had commented that one has to achieve perfection 100% of the time if one is to consistently achieve success.

Small changes in the setting of the Phaco instrument can lead to significant changes to the corneal endothelium. Ultrasound modulation techniques and the conservation of dispersed energy are true goals to achieve if one is to aim for the perfection of a virtually untouched eye at the end of the procedure.

Perhaps the outstanding characteristic of this book is the author's ability to select critically the various nuances of the machine vis-a-vis the applicability for an individual procedure. I am proud and excited to be asked to contribute the foreword and I am sure this book will be regarded as an outstanding contribution to the field of cataract removal.

Prof Keiki R Mehta
Surgical Director and Chief, Dr Keiki Mehta International Eye Institute
Professor Emeritus, Dr DY Patil Medical College, Bombay University, Mumbai
Emeritus Consultant Ophthalmologist, Breach Candy Hospital, Mumbai
Past President and Chairman Scientific of the All India Ophthalmologists Association
Past President, Indian Intraocular Implant and Refractive Society
Chairman, Iconic Eye Advance Congresses for last 28 years
Honorary Ophthalmic Surgeon to
The Governor of Maharashtra, Maharashtra Police and
Armed Forces, Government of India
Awarded Padmashree in recognition of his services to Indian ophthalmology in 2008

Preface

I have written three books on Phacoemulsification surgery.

My first book "Simplified Phacoemulsification" gives an idea about how to perform Phacoemulsification surgery.

"Text and Atlas Slit Lamp Biomicroscopy for Assessment in Cataract Surgery" gives information about how to examine the patient before surgery.

"Do's & Don'ts in Phaco Surgery—Text and Atlas" gives an idea about the analysis of our own surgical steps.

After writing these three books, I had a strong inclination to write something new which will assist surgeons to do better Phaco surgery.

I have been conducting the cataract training program since 2002 and I have noticed that even after the successful completion of Phaco training, the surgeons are always in a dilemma how to set parameters of Phaco machine in different situations of cataract.

This frequently asked question from doctors has given motivation to write a book on "*Phaco Machine and its Applications.*"

Sharing the knowledge is my main purpose which I have learnt from my mother Chand Toshniwal. My father, Dr Sham Toshniwal, taught from the beginning of practice that surgery is not only just the skill of a surgeon but also a combination of good operation theater and atmosphere, well-trained nursing team, good quality of instruments, and knowledge of machine which is concerned with the surgical procedures and helpful for a better surgical outcome. All these together will definitely increase the confidence of work.

Being mindful of the wisdom bestowed by my parents and doubts of many doctors motivated me to write this unique book.

In this book, information related to parts of Phaco machine (hardware, software), definitions and description of parameters, use of parameters for all steps of Phaco surgery, application of parameters for a different variety of cataracts in the form of charts, and some tips related to troubleshooting in machine have been introduced.

The idea of making this book is that surgeons can carry it easily with them to the operation theater and refer to set the proper parameters with respect to that particular case.

I strongly feel that such a kind of distinctive and user-oriented book on Phaco machine will be definitely helpful to provide good knowledge for betterment of Phaco surgery. It will be helpful to the doctors worldwide.

Navneet Toshniwal

Acknowledgments

First and foremost, I am grateful to the Almighty God that I thought to write a book on Phaco machine.

I am grateful for the blessings of my father, Dr Sham Toshniwal, who was a guide and mentor to me throughout my academic career, and my mother, Chand Toshniwal, who says "Give your knowledge to all. It will increase more and more only by giving." These motivational words inspired me to share my experiences in the form of books. "Thanks" is a very short word for them.

I am also grateful to the world-famous renowned ophthalmologist Padmashree Dr Keiki Mehta from Mumbai, who is one of the pioneer of Phaco surgery in India. He has inspired me in my academic career through his presentations and lectures at state, national, and international conferences. Special thanks and gratitude to him for writing the Foreword for this book.

I would like to mention the name of my wife and life partner Sunita who often accompanies me to many international conferences. In such conferences, many doctors have suggested this topic to me but it was Sunita who insisted and was the real force behind me writing this book.

I would also like to thanks my uncle, Dr Murli Toshniwal, my brother Dr Nitin and Dr Kirti Toshniwal; sister Dr Neeta and Dr Nilesh Bhandari who always supports me. They have always encouraged and motivated me throughout this journey. I also thank my sister-in-law Rekha Rathi from Aurangabad and cousins Kanhaiyalal, Sanjay, all Toshniwal family members who always support me.

Thanks are due to Dr Rucha Kothadia (ophthalmologist), Dr Vikram Hirekerur, Mr Ram Adnak (optometrist), and Dr Richa Kamble who have played an important role in completion of this book.

I thanks my elder son Dr Nikhil who is doing cornea fellowship at Sankara Nethralaya, Chennai; daughter-in-law Dr Ayushi who is doing PG at the Medical College Baroda, SSG Hospital, Vadodara, Gujarat and my younger son Dr Sumit and nephew Dr Amit. They have helped a lot in the editing of this book. I am also thankful to a nephew Naitik Bhandari who has helped me for the front cover of this book.

I would like to extend my special thanks to Mr Jitendar P Vij (Group Chairman), Mr Ankit Vij (Managing Director), Mr MS Mani (Group President), Ms Chetna Malhotra Vohra (Associate Director—Content Strategy), Ms Pooja Bhandari (Production Head), Ruby Sharma (Project Manager), Nikita Chauhan (Senior Development Editor), Saima Rashid (Publishing Manager) and all concerned team members of Jaypee Brothers Medical Publishers, New Delhi, India, for helping me in making of this book.

I also thank Dr Kishor Babar and all the team of Navneet Hospital, Solapur, Maharashtra, India.

I would like to specially thank all the doctors who have trained at our hospital. Their suggestions and motivation were really helpful for this work.

Last, but not the least, my special thanks and gratitude are due toward all the patients. It is because of the that we are in this noble profession.

Contents

Chapter 1: Introduction — 1
About this Book 1

Chapter 2: Components of Phaco Machine — 2
Parts of Phaco Machine 2
Key Points 12

Chapter 3: Energy — 13
Definition 13
Principle 13
Longitudinal Phaco (Traditional Phaco) 13
Types of Delivery System of Energy 14
Different Modes of Energy 14
Modified Modes of Energy 23
Combination of Longitudinal and Transverse Forms of Energy 26
Key Points 27

Chapter 4: Vacuum — 28
Principle 28
Uses of Vacuum 29
Different Settings of Vacuum 29
Delivery System of Vacuum 33
Key Points 34

Chapter 5: Aspiration Flow Rate — 35
Principle 35
Uses 35
Different Settings of Flow Rate 36
Key Points 39

Chapter 6: Association of Energy Vacuum and Flow Rate — 40
Important Factors Related to Association of Energy, Vacuum, and Flow Rate 40
Key Points 45

Chapter 7: Torsional Technology — 46
Principle 46
Advantages 46

Machine Features 47
Surgical Parameters 50
Disadvantages 54
Centurion Vision System 54
Key Points 55

Chapter 8: Phaco Parameters in Different Types of Cataract   56
Modes 56
Parameters in the Form of Chart 57
Key Points 68

Chapter 9: Troubleshooting   69
Difficulties Occurring during Surgery 69
Key Points 74

Chapter 10: Selection of Phaco Machine   75
Prerequisites 75
Key Points 76

Instruments Invented by Dr Navneet Toshniwal   77
Index   79

CHAPTER 1

Introduction

One should know in details about the Phaco machine to do better Phaco surgery.

Surgeons are dependent on technical people from the company to understand these parameters in the initial days of Phaco practice.

It takes quite a long time to understand these parameters used in the surgery.

Most important aim to write on this subject is to decrease the learning curve to understand the Phaco machine.

ABOUT THIS BOOK

- Definition and principle of all the components and parameters of the Phaco machine have been explained in a simple way.
- Implementation of these parameters in the surgical steps is mentioned in practical way.
- Parameters mentioned are not always same, but it can be customized from surgeon to surgeon and case to case related to variable anatomy.
- Separate chapter is written on parameters related to different varieties of cataracts.
- Surgeon can set these parameters according to their knowledge and surgical experience.
- Do not think to change these parameters frequently in normal cataract cases.
- To start with, selection of ideal cases to implement these parameters is very important factor to understand the Phaco machine in a better way.
- Chapter on parameters should be read lastly.
- Many times, it is mentioned panel/linear, which means that first choice is to set the parameters in panel.

CHAPTER 2

Components of Phaco Machine

INTRODUCTION

- Phaco surgery is based on the following aspects:
  - Concept of Phaco
  - Knowing about Phaco machine
- Phaco surgery is a machine-dependent surgery.
- One should know one's own Phaco machine in a simple way, which is an integral part of a successful Phaco surgery.
- Understanding the Phaco machine needs adequate time.
- When you start working with Phaco machine, you understand different features of Phaco machine and its scientific use for better surgery with less complication rate.
- It is like any other machine or car; as you use or drive it more and more, you will understand more salient features.

PARTS OF PHACO MACHINE

- Basic console with screen
- Pump
- Tubing set
- Foot pedal
- Phaco probe
- Irrigation and aspiration (I/A) cannula
- Irrigation stand
- Diathermy
- Vitrectomy cutter

Basic Console with Screen

- It contains basic hardware and software of machine.
- All the settings of parameters such as energy, vacuum, aspiration flow rate, diathermy, vitrectomy, and their details are displayed on the screen.
- Continuous irrigation switch is an important option.
- There is a switch for automated operation of irrigation stand.

- Remote control is also provided with many machines, which are with wire or wireless.
- Screen has either touch button or screen touch facility.

Pump

Three types of pump are present:
1. Diaphragmatic pump
2. Venturi pump
3. Peristaltic pump

Diaphragmatic Pump

Principle:
- It has flexible membrane to generate the vacuum.
- With this pump, vacuum reaches to preset level without occlusion.

Advantages:
- Hold and chop of nucleus is quick and strong.
- Easy removal of small pieces of nucleus

Disadvantage:
- Safety margin of surgical steps is less.

Venturi Pump

Principle:
- Compressed gas creates negative suction force inside a closed chamber, which is directly transmitted to handpiece.
- Vacuum and aspiration flow rate are working together in this pump.

Advantages:
- Surgical procedure is fast.
- Holding capacity of tissue is better, as vacuum works more efficiently.

Disadvantages:
- Safety margin of surgical steps is less.
- Catching and chaffing of iris can occur.
- Catching of posterior capsule can occur.

Peristaltic Pump

It is the most commonly used pump in Phaco practice.

Principle:
Rotation of rollers by the pump pinches the soft silicon tubing, which creates negative pressure by squeezing the fluid out of the tube.

In this system, vacuum is built up only when the tip gets occluded.

Components of Phaco Machine

Features:
- Energy, vacuum and aspiration flow rate work independently but assist each other.
- Correlation of energy, vacuum and flow rate in steps of nucleus management, I/A of cortex and epinucleus is the most important learning point.
- One should know the correct parameters of energy, vacuum and flow rate.
- Different modulations concerned with energy, vacuum and flow rate can be understood step by step with practice.
- Once one will have the theoretical as well as practical knowledge about Phaco machine, then use of Phaco parameters related to surgical steps is very easy.

Advantages:
- It is safe.
- Complicated cases can be handled in a safe and skillful way.
- Level of confidence of workup is better.
- Chances of catching iris and capsule are less.

Disadvantage:
- Speed of surgical procedure is relatively adequate or less.

In some machines, both the peristaltic and venturi pumps work together.

Tubing Set
- Phaco probe is attached to the Phaco machine with tubing.
- Prime and tuning of machine are important to start the machine.
- In higher end machines, one can get presterile pouch of tubing which is called cassette.
- Phaco fluidics depends upon the quality of tubing.
- These tubings are made up of silicon materials which are disposable or nondisposable.

Tubing
- *Disposable*

  Advantages:
  - Irrigation flow is good.
  - Functioning of vacuum and aspiration flow rate, i.e., Phaco fluidics is better.
  - Due to new tubing, chances of infection are less.

  Disadvantage:
  - It is expensive.

- *Nondisposable*
  Advantages:
  - Tubing can be used repeatedly.
  - It can be autoclaved.
  - It can be ethylene oxide (ETO) sterilized.
  - It is cost-effective.

  Disadvantages:
  - Sometimes, repeated use of tubing decreases the efficiency of Phaco fluidics.
  - There is a chance of infection.

When to stop using these tubings?
These tubings should stop, when:
- The color gets faint. Yellow color indicates old tubing.
- Phaco fluidics is not appropriate.
- Hard consistency of tubing indicates less flexibility.
- Ends of tubing get roughened.
- There is a leakage in the tubing.
- There is a mechanical damage.

Maintenance of tubing:
Cleaning of tubing is an art:
- Cleaning is done by balanced salt solution (BSS)
- Followed by cleaning twice with distilled water.
- Most important point is to make the tubing completely dry before sterilization.

Keeping the Phaco probe with autoclavable tubing in the Phaco tray is an art, which can increase the life of Phaco probe and tubing.

Foot Pedal

- Learning the foot pedal is very important in the beginning of Phaco practice. It is like learning the accelerator of the car.
- Different modes and sub-modes in steps of Phaco, I/A, diathermy, and vitrectomy are controlled by foot pedal.
- One can program two lateral side switches of foot pedal to change the sub-modes.
- Continuous irrigation is also controlled by foot pedal.

Principle

Three positions work in a foot pedal (**Fig. 1**):
- There are audible and tactile sensations to detect position of foot pedal.
- The placement of foot pedal on the flooring should be comfortable for the surgeon.

Components of Phaco Machine

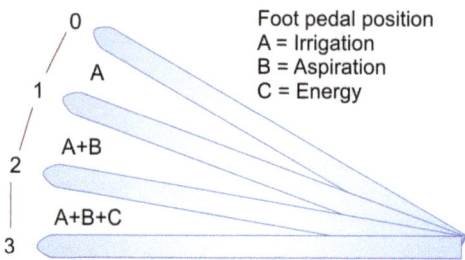

Fig. 1: Foot pedal position. 1. Position A is irrigation, 2. Position B is irrigation and aspiration, 3. Position C is irrigation, aspiration, and energy.

- *Degree of travel or gap among these three positions of foot pedal (foot position threshold) can be customized.*

Reflux

This is the unique feature present in the foot pedal.

The basic principle is repulsion of structures such as iris and posterior capsule which has been accidently caught in the aspiration port.

Phaco Probe and Its Accessories

Phaco Probe

Principle:
- It is a piezoelectric substance which converts electronic energy into ultrasound energy for emulsification of nucleus under the influence of electrical signal.

Features:
- Frequency ranges from 30,000 to 60,000 Hz. Most commonly used is 40,000 Hz.
- Frequency is fixed for that particular probe.
- Different probes have different piezoelectric crystals ranging from two to four in number.
- Stroke length is a to-and-fro movement of Phaco tip which emulsifies the tissue in front of the tip.
- Stroke length varies with percentage of energy.

Phaco probe should be:
- Light weight
- Handy
- Not too long or not too short
- Piezoelectric crystals are more important. If it is more in number, then efficiency is more.
- Design of Phaco probe should be in such a way that—it should have a good grip.

Accessories
- Phaco tip
- Sleeve
- Wrench

Phaco tip:
- Straight
- Angulated (Kelman)

Distal end of Phaco tip is having angulation from 0 to 45° (**Table 1**).

Table 1: Correlation of Phaco tip angulation with its effect on hold and cutting of nucleus.

Degree	Figure	Hold	Cutting
0		+++	---
15		++	+
30		+	++
45		---	+++

According to the author, degree means effect.
It means that 0° effect will hold the nucleus better and 45° effect will cut the nucleus better.

- *Straight tip:*
  This is commonly used tip in practice (**Fig. 2**).
  Features:
  - There is no angulation in the tip.
  - Angulation of distal end of Phaco tip varies from 0 to 45°.

  Advantages:
  - Using this tip is easy for every surgeon in the initial days of practice.
  - Entry of Phaco tip through the incision is easy.
  - In nucleus management, hold and chop step is better with this tip.

Straight tip

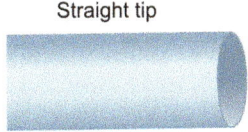

Fig. 2: Straight tip.

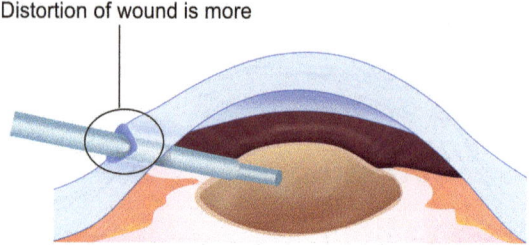

Fig. 3: Distortion of incision due to straight tip.

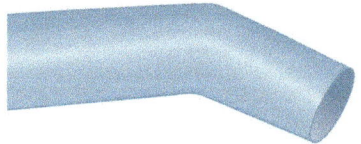

Fig. 4: Angulated tip (Kelman).

Disadvantages:
- As the plane of entry (incision) and plane of working (level of nucleus) are different, incision can get distorted due to this tip (**Fig. 3**).

Distortion will lead to:
- Wound leak
- Shallow anterior chamber
- Injury to cornea, iris, anterior and posterior capsule

This distortion is more in:
- Deep socket
- Deep anterior chamber
- Deep bag
- High myopia
- Hypotony

Features such as torsional technology are not possible with straight tip.
- *Angulated tip (Kelman)* (**Fig. 4**):

Features:
- Tip is angulated.
- Angulation of distal end of Phaco tip varies from 0 to 45°.
- Generally 30° or 45° tip is used.
- There are different designs of distal end of the Kelman tip such as Cobra tip, Round tip, and Mini-flared tip.

Advantages:
Due to angulation of tip, working plane is near to nuclear plane automatically, thus distortion of incision is less during nucleus management (**Fig. 5**).
- Trench is easy to perform.

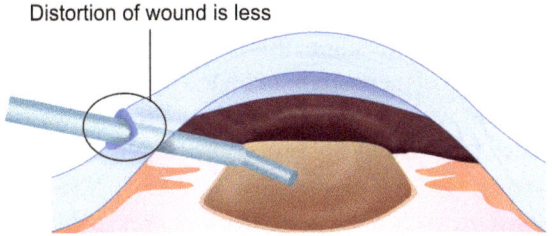

Fig. 5: Distortion of wound.

- Stability of anterior chamber is better.
- Torsional technology and ellipsoid technology can be used easily which has high cutting efficiency and is very helpful in hard cataract.

Disadvantages:
- Entry and removal of Phaco tip through the wound need practice.
- It can touch iris during entry or removal of Phaco tip.
- Hold and lift half part of the nucleus after division is relatively difficult in stop and chop technique.
- During removal of pieces due to angulation, one can take precaution of avoiding damage to posterior capsule.
- Understanding the direction of Phaco tip with respect to nucleus during nucleus management is a learning process.
- Use of this tip is relatively difficult in shallow anterior chamber, shallow bag, etc.

Gauge and inner diameter of the tip:
- 19 gauge: 1.1-mm diameter
- 20 gauge: 0.9-mm diameter
- 21 gauge: 0.7-mm diameter

Commonly used gauge is 19 or 20.

Other types of Phaco tip:
- Mackool tip
- Flared tip
- Aspiration bypass system (ABS) tip
- Barrett's micro-flow tip
- Cobra tip
- Diaphragm tip
- Turbo Sonics tip

Sleeve:
Phaco tip is surrounded by sleeve.

Uses:
- Irrigating flow is very well controlled by sleeve.
- Direction of sleeve with holes regulates water current in eye.

Components of Phaco Machine

- Generally, sleeve with holes is placed horizontally when Phaco tip is in bevel-up or bevel-down position, this is basic position of sleeve.
- During trench in bevel up position of Phaco tip, sleeve is adjusted in such a way that flow of water current is horizontal for better visualization of depth of groove throughout the procedure. *It assists separation of layers of lens too.*
- *During removal of pieces of nucleus, sleeve is adjusted in such a way that flow of water current is horizontal which assists the Phaco fluidics.*

Advantages:
- It protects the energy transmission from tip.
- It helps to maintain architecture of incision.

Exposure of Phaco tip with respect to sleeve depends upon many factors such as:
- Hard cataract → More exposed tip
- Soft cataract → Less exposed tip
- Shallow AC → Less exposed tip
- Small pupil → Less exposed tip
- Hazy cornea → Less exposed tip
- Floppy iris → Less exposed tip

Important fact:
Size of incision is not dependent on size of Phaco tip, but it depends on thickness of sleeve.
Different thickness of sleeve is identified by color of sleeve:
- Purple
- Pink
- Yellow
- Blue
- Light blue
- White
- Clear
- Orange

When to change the sleeve?
The sleeve is changed when:
- It gets torn
- There is change of color
- Strength gets reduced

Material used:
High-quality silicon material is used.

Advantage:
Architecture of incision is maintained during I/A procedure.

Wrench:
- Wrench is used to tighten *Phaco* tip to *Phaco* probe.
- It can be made up of steel or titanium.
- It can be autoclaved or ETO sterilization.
- Different designs of wrench for different machines

Irrigation and Aspiration Cannula

Irrigation and aspiration step is for removal of epinucleus, cortex, and very soft nucleus.
Materials used are:
- Metal
- Silicon

Types of Cannula
- Coaxial cannula
- Bimanual cannula

Coaxial cannula:
- Coaxial I/A cannula is working through main port incision.
- In coaxial I/A, tip is used with sleeve.

Role of sleeve in I/A:
During irrigation aspiration, working plane is beneath the anterior capsule. Cannula is placed horizontally and sleeve can be adjusted in such a way that horizontal flow of water current, which actually assists to loosen the epinucleus and cortex, identifies the mass of tissue as a bulk or apex which will be helpful for procedure.

In other words, if direction of high-flow water current is at different plane, this may hit iris posteriorly which can constrict the pupil.

Hassle-free entry of I/A cannula with sleeve depends on adjustment of sleeve with respect to cannula.

Shape of tips:
- Straight
- Curved, generally 45°
- J shape

Bimanual cannula:
- Two different cannulas are used separately for I/A.
- Irrigation port is having two sideway holes at the distal end of the tip.
- Aspiration port is having one hole in the center at the distal end of the tip.
- These cannulas are generally passed through side port incision.
- These cannulas are without sleeve.

Irrigation Stand
- Flow of irrigation depends on the height of irrigation stand.
- It is manual or automated.
- Generally, bottle height is kept at 110 cm and varies according to different situations.

Diathermy
- This is digital diathermy.
- Cauterization of the blood vessel is smooth.
- There is no contracture of the scleral tissue in limbal incision.
- There are less chances of postcautery astigmatism.
- Generally, parameter of diathermy is kept from 20 to 40%.

Vitrectomy Cutter
- Vitrectomy cutter is supplied with Phaco machine, which is used for anterior and mid vitrectomy only.
- Set of vitrectomy should be kept ready before every Phaco procedure and especially where surgeon expects posterior capsule rupture in conditions such as posterior polar cataract, hard cataract, subluxated cataract, cataract with pseudoexfoliation, and traumatic cataract.
- One should know the principle and procedure of vitrectomy.
- Detailed knowledge of parameters of anterior vitrectomy procedure is important.
- Cutting rate should be as high as possible.
- Vacuum and flow rate should be adequate and adjusted according to the situation.

Parameters
Generally used parameters are as follows:
- Irrigating fluid: Low bottle height
- Cutting rate: 600–2,500 cuts per minute (cpm)
- Flow rate: 20–26 cc/min
- Vacuum: 150–250 mm Hg

Flow rate and vacuum can be kept panel/linear.
These parameters can be varied according to the situation.

KEY POINTS
- One should know one's own Phaco machine in a simple way which is an integral part of successful Phaco surgery.
- Like every machine, knowledge of parts or components of Phaco machine is helpful in doing Phaco surgery with confidence.
- Prime, tune, and cleaning of the machine are important factors.

CHAPTER 3

Energy

DEFINITION
Energy is defined as the ability to emulsify the nucleus.

PRINCIPLE
Emulsification of nucleus is in the following ways:
- *Jackhammer effect*:
  - It is the direct mechanical impact on the nucleus to emulsify it.
- *Cavitational effect*:
  - This is a highly effective source of emulsification.
  - High-frequency vibration of needle and acoustic wave form tiny air bubbles.
  - These tiny air bubbles induce localized implosion on nuclear material for better emulsification.
- *Acoustic wave of fluid*:
  - It is like wave of ocean, generated by the forward movements of the tip which can disintegrate the lens material.

INTRODUCTION
Energy is one of the important parameters of Phaco machine.
- Energy is delivered by Phaco probe.
- It is ultrasound energy.
- Energy is used to emulsify the hard part of cataract, i.e., nucleus.
- Sometimes, energy is used to emulsify thick or sticky epinucleus.
- As energy can burn cornea or iris during Phaco, one should have an overall idea about parameters used in all steps of nucleus management.
- One should know the different modes and delivery system of energy used for Phaco.

LONGITUDINAL PHACO (TRADITIONAL PHACO)
This is the most commonly used ultrasound energy.

Stroke Length

- It is the distance by which the Phaco tip moves to and fro.
- It can be altered by changing the Phaco power.
- More energy means more stroke length, i.e., more area of emulsification of nucleus ahead of the Phaco tip.

Frequency

- It is the number of times the Phaco tip moves.
- It is fixed for every Phaco handpiece.
- It is measured in kHz.

TYPES OF DELIVERY SYSTEM OF ENERGY

Linear

This is a gradual rise in the energy from zero to preset level in a linear way as foot pedal is pressed.

Panel

This is sudden rise in the energy from zero to preset level as soon as foot pedal is pressed.

DIFFERENT MODES OF ENERGY

- *Continuous energy*
- *Pulse*
- *Hyperpulse*
- *Short pulse*
- *Long pulse*
- *Low-power pulse*
- *High-power pulse*
- *Single burst*
- *Multiburst*
- *Continuous burst*

Continuous Energy

- It is the continuous form of energy (**Fig. 1**).
- There is no off time.

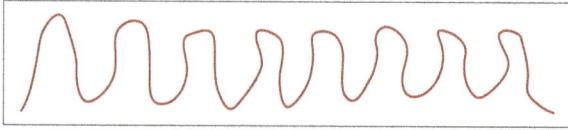

Fig. 1: Continuous energy.

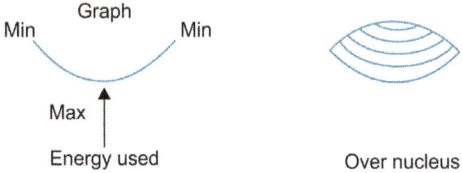

Fig. 2: Trench.

It can be linear or panel.

Linear

- Energy used is from 0 to 100.
- It is a commonly used form of energy.
- As the foot pedal is pressed, it will gradually increase.
- It is controlled energy.

Indications:
Trench (Fig. 2):
- Continuous linear mode is the most important form of energy used for trench.
- Hardness of nucleus varies from one end to the other and anterior to posterior.
- Energy can be set according to the hardness of nucleus.
- Energy used minimum to start with, maximum in the center, and then minimum to complete the trench

Parameters:
- Generally 60–80% energy is used for trench.
- In hard cataract, it can be set to 70–80% or more.
- In soft cataract, it can be decreased 60–70% or less.

Division:
After trench, one can separate or divide the nucleus either mechanically or sometimes can hold (engage) the half mass of nucleus with Phaco tip and then divide with chopper.

Parameter:
Generally, 20–50% energy is used.

Hold and chop:
- Continuous linear mode is the most important form of energy for hold.
- In this step, not only hold but also maintaining the hold is important.
- Needs adequate energy to embed in the mass.

Parameter:
Generally, 20–50% energy is used.

Panel
- As the foot pedal is pressed, energy reaches to the preset level suddenly.
- Energy used in panel is called "burst mode."

Indications:
- It can be used in trench, hold and chop, and direct chop step of nucleus management.
- In very hard cataract, one can set 70% energy during trench; it means tissue will emulsify with same energy from start to end point. Subsequently, 40–50% of energy can be used for hold and chop.
- For direct chop technique in hard cataract, this mode of energy is helpful.

Disadvantages:
- Turbulence in anterior chamber
- Consumption of energy is more.
- Wound burn

Pulse Energy

- Energy used in pulses (**Fig. 3**)
- This form of energy has cutting and holding ability.
- Controlled way of emulsification of nucleus
- Energy transferred in the eye is less.
- Generally, it is used in linear mode.

Indications:
- Removal of small pieces of nucleus
- This mode of energy is used sometimes in grades I and II cataract for hold and lift of nucleus before chop for which energy can be set according to the hardness of nucleus.

Chatter means repulsion of nucleus; it occurs if energy is used more than needed.

Hyperpulse Energy

*This is new modulation of energy to overcome all disadvantages of traditional energy (**Fig. 4**).*
- On and off time is fixed.

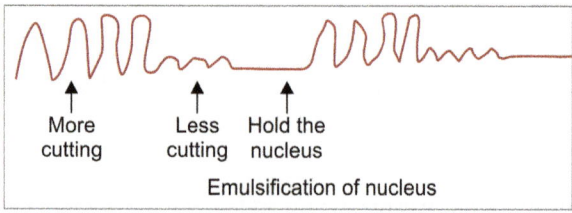

Fig. 3: Pulse energy.

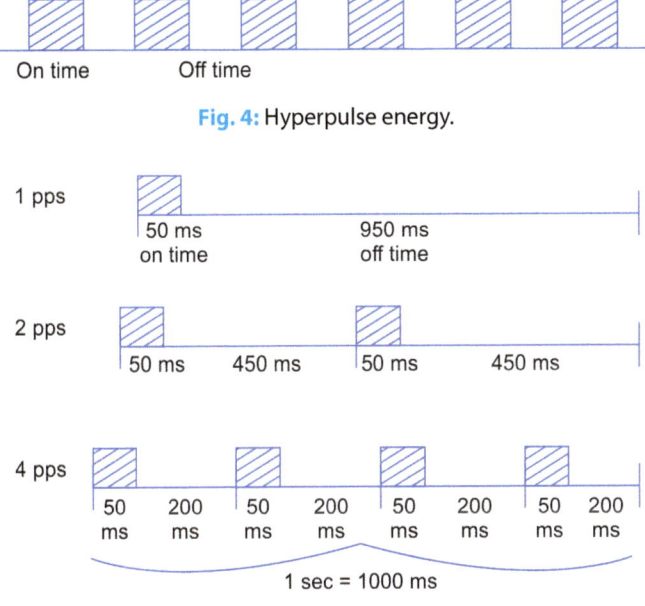

Fig. 4: Hyperpulse energy.

Fig. 5: Short pulse. (PPS: pulse per second)

- On time is for emulsification of nucleus.
- Off time is for hold of nucleus.
- Energy consumption is less without compromising the cutting efficiency of nucleus.

There are different types of modification in hyperpulse, where on time is fixed and off time is variable.

Short Pulse (Fig. 5; Table 1)

Introduction:
- 50 ms on time is fixed.
- Off time is variable.
- Short pulses can be set from 1 to 14 pps.

Parameters:
- Commonly used parameters are 6 pps.
- Delivery of energy is linear.

Indications:
- For removal of small pieces of nucleus
- For removal of last pieces of nucleus
- In soft cataract:
  - In stop and chop technique, after nucleus division for hold and lift of half part of nucleus

Table 1: Chart of short pulse.

PPS (pulses per second)	Calculation	On time (ms)	Off time (ms)
1	1,000 ÷ 1 = 1,000	50	950
2	1,000 ÷ 2 = 500	50	450
3	1,000 ÷ 3 = 333	50	283
4	1,000 ÷ 4 = 250	50	200
5	1,000 ÷ 5 = 200	50	150
6	1,000 ÷ 6 = 166	50	116
7	1,000 ÷ 7 = 142	50	92
8	1,000 ÷ 8 = 125	50	75
9	1,000 ÷ 9 = 111	50	61
10	1,000 ÷ 10 = 100	50	50
11	1,000 ÷ 11 = 90	50	40
12	1,000 ÷ 12 = 83	50	33
13	1,000 ÷ 13 = 76	50	26
14	1,000 ÷ 14 = 71	50	21

1 s = 1,000 ms

- Hold, lift, and emulsification of complete nucleus after hydrodelineation
- For removal of epinucleus

Advantages:
- Due to more off time, pieces come toward the Phaco tip easily, i.e., better followability.
- It is safe for cornea as on time is less.
- It is a safe mode for removal of last pieces of nucleus to avoid PCR.

Long Pulse (Fig. 6; Table 2)

Introduction:
- 150 ms of on time is fixed.
- Off time is variable.
- Long pulses can be set from 1 to 6.

Parameters:
- Commonly used parameters are 4 pps.
- Delivery of energy is linear.

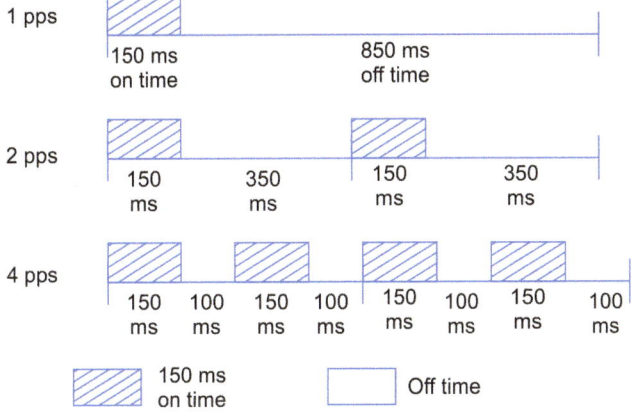

Fig. 6: Long pulse. (pps: pulse per second)

PPS (pulses per second)	Calculation	On time (ms)	Off time (ms)
1	1,000 ÷ 1 = 1,000	150	850
2	1,000 ÷ 2 = 500	150	350
3	1,000 ÷ 3 = 333	150	183
4	1,000 ÷ 4 = 250	150	100
5	1,000 ÷ 5 = 200	150	50
6	1,000 ÷ 6 = 166	150	16

Table 2: Chart of long pulse.

1 s = 1,000 ms

Indications:
For removal of small pieces of nucleus:
- In hard cataract, for removal of small pieces of nucleus, one can use the parameters from 2 to 4 pps.
- In soft cataract, for removal of small pieces of nucleus, one can use the parameters from 1 to 2 pps.

For hold and lift of nucleus:
- In grades III and IV cataract, parameters used are 4–6 pps.
- In soft cataract, parameters used are 2–4 pps.

For epinucleus:
In thick epinucleus or in sticky epinucleus cataract, one can use this mode with 1 pps or 2 pps.

20 Energy

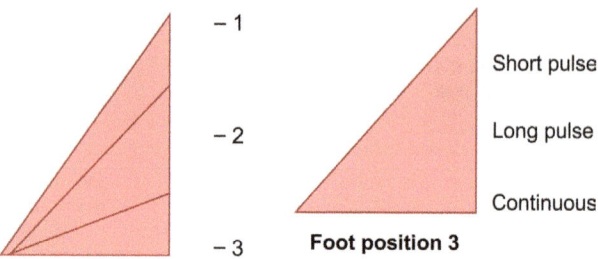

Fig. 7: Low-power pulse.

Advantages:
- Due to on and off time, followability of the nuclear pieces is better.
- Chances of corneal burn and PCR are less.

Low-power Pulse

Introduction:
- This energy mode is working in foot pedal position 3.
- Foot pedal position 3 is divided into three compartments from top to bottom. As you press the foot pedal, it will start working as short pulse, then in mid-phase as long pulse and when you press completely, it works as a continuous mode of energy **(Fig. 7)**.
- It means that the duration of energy is gradually increasing from a small duration of 50 ms, then 150 ms, and then works as a continuous mode.

Indications:
Low-power pulse works in the following ways:
- In removal of small pieces of nucleus:
  - Short pulses for soft part of nucleus
  - Long pulses for relatively hard part of nucleus
  - Continuous mode of energy used to hold and chop the big pieces during removal of small pieces
- In hold and chop of nucleus

This mode of energy is used for grades II to IV cataract.

Advantages:
Surgeon can hold, chop, and remove the small pieces simultaneously with this single mode of energy. So, there is no need to change the parameters in between the steps.
- Adequate energy for adequate purpose
- This mode can be used for normal cataract, soft cataract, and hard cataract too.

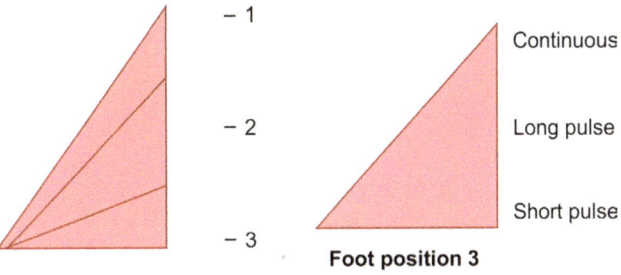

Fig. 8: High-power pulse.

High-power Pulse

Introduction:
- This energy mode is working in foot pedal position 3.
- Foot pedal position 3 is divided into three compartments from top to bottom. As you press the foot pedal, it will start working as a continuous mode of energy, then in mid-phase long pulse and when you press completely, it works as a short pulse (**Fig. 8**).

Indications:
This unique power modulation works in the following way:
- *In hold and chop of nucleus*:
  - Continuous energy is to bury the Phaco tip in mass.
  - Long pulse will be helpful to maintain the hold before chop.
- *In removal of small pieces of nucleus*:
  - Long pulse and short pulse are important applications for removal of small pieces.
- *Direct chop technique*:
  - It can be used in this technique in a unique way.

In such type of modulation, energy can be used in burst mode.

Advantages:
- Energy used in panel is called a burst mode.
- It is safe for the last pieces of nucleus removal.
- Hold, chop, and removal of small pieces of nucleus can occur with this one mode, so there is no need to change the parameters in between steps.

Single Burst (Fig. 9)

- Energy used in panel is called a burst mode.
- Single burst means 110 ms is on time and 890 ms is off time.
- If energy is kept at 40%, then it means that 40% energy will work for 110 ms in one cycle.

22 Energy

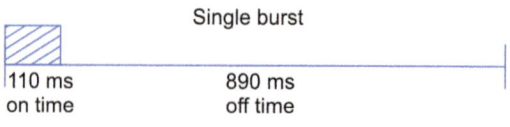

Fig. 9: Single burst.

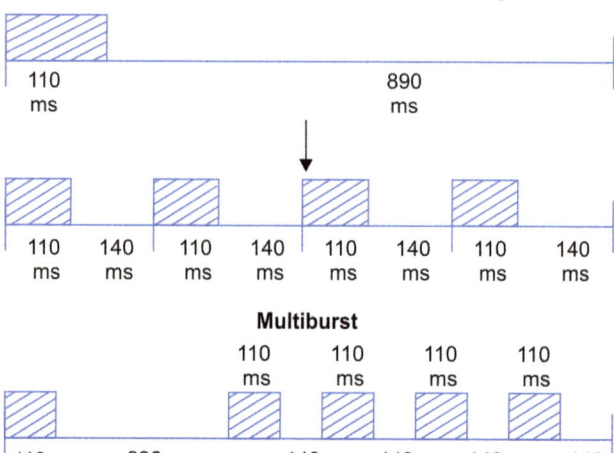

Fig. 10: Multiburst.

Indications:
- For removal of pieces of nucleus in hard cataract
- Sometimes, it is helpful for hold and chop in hard cataract

Multiburst (Fig. 10)
- One single burst gradually increases to four bursts per second as foot pedal is pressed.
- It means that single burst followed by four bursts in one cycle.
- Single burst means 110 ms on time and 890 ms off time.
- Four bursts in one cycle mean on time is 110 ms and off time is 140 ms.

Indications

This mode of energy is helpful for hard cataract.
- *In stop and chop technique:*
  - For hold and chop
  - For removal of pieces
- *In direct chop technique*

Continuous Burst

As you press the foot pedal, it starts working as single burst; in mid-phase, it works as multiburst and it works as a continuous burst of energy.

Indications

This mode of energy is generally used in hard or very hard cataract.
- *Stop and chop technique*:
  Trench:
  - First few strokes are continuous burst and last few strokes can be used in linear mode.

  Hold and chop and removal of small pieces of nucleus:
  - Continuous mode can be used for hold and chop and single and multiple bursts can be used in removal of small pieces.
- *Direct chop technique*

This mode of energy can be used for hard cataract.

MODIFIED MODES OF ENERGY

- Whitestar
- Variable Whitestar

Whitestar

- It is combination of on time and off time which is variable.
- It can be customized for optimum use of continuous form of energy.
- Functioning of Whitestar is based on duty cycle.

Duty Cycle (**Table 3**)

- 1,000 ms of continuous power
- Micropulse division
- On time and off time can be customized.
- On and off time varies from 2 to 32 ms.
- Ratio of Phaco on time to total (or cycle) time is expressed as percentage.

How to calculate duty cycle:
It can be calculated alphabetically:
- C means → 3 × 2 = 6
- B means → 2 × 2 = 4
- D means → 4 × 2 = 8
- F means → 6 × 2 = 12
- N means → 14 × 2 = 28
- L means → 12 × 2 = 24
- I means → 9 × 2 = 18

Example:

		On time	Off time
DB	→	8	4

$$\frac{8}{8+4} \rightarrow 8/12 = 67\% \text{ on time}$$

		On time	Off time
BD	→	4	8

$$\frac{4}{4+8} \rightarrow 4/12 = 33\% \text{ on time}$$

Table 3: Duty cycle chart.

	On time	Off time	Calculation: On time ÷ (On time + Off time)	On time
CN	6	28	6 ÷ (6 + 28) = 6 ÷ 34	18%
CL	6	24	6 ÷ (6 + 24) = 6 ÷ 30	20%
BL	4	24	4 ÷ (4 + 24) = 4 ÷ 28	14%
DI	8	18	8 ÷ (8 + 18) = 8 ÷ 26	31%
CI	6	18	6 ÷ (6 + 18) = 6 ÷ 24	25%
CF	6	12	6 ÷ (6 + 12) = 6 ÷ 18	33%
CD	6	8	6 ÷ (6 + 8) = 6 ÷ 14	43%
BD	4	8	4 ÷ (4 + 8) = 4 ÷ 12	33%
DB	8	4	8 ÷ (8 + 4) = 8 ÷ 12	67%
CB	6	4	6 ÷ (6 + 4) = 6 ÷ 10	60%

Indications:
This mode of energy can be used for all steps of nucleus management.
- This different form of energy is used for trench when you will increase on time at the highest, i.e., 30-2.
- Due to variation in on time, it can be used for hold and chop step for all grades of cataract.
- Due to variation in off time, followability is better during removal of small pieces.

This module is having more advantage for hold and chop and removal of small pieces; it is especially safe for last pieces also.

Advantages:
- All the advantages of this mode are purely based on customization of on and off time.
  - Customization of on time is for emulsification of nucleus.
  - Customization of off time is for hold of nucleus.
- In this mode of energy, although cutting efficiency is better but chances of corneal burn are less.

- Magnetic followability of the nuclear pieces is noticed during removal of small pieces.
- Due to variation in on and off time, it is also safe for last pieces removal.
- This can be superimposed on other forms of power modulations such as:
  - Short pulse
  - Long pulse
  - Burst mode
  - Low-power pulse
  - High-power pulse
  - Continuous mode

Variable Whitestar

- It is a very unique type of energy modulation.
- *It is a continuous linear form of energy and can be customized.*
- In foot position 3, energy can be used in an ascending or a descending way.
- Energy used in an ascending way is called variable Whitestar 1 (**Fig. 11A**).
- Energy used in a descending way is called variable Whitestar 2 (**Fig. 11B**).

Advantages

- This mode of energy can be used for all grades of cataract.
- This mode is helpful in hold and chop and removal of pieces step of nucleus management.

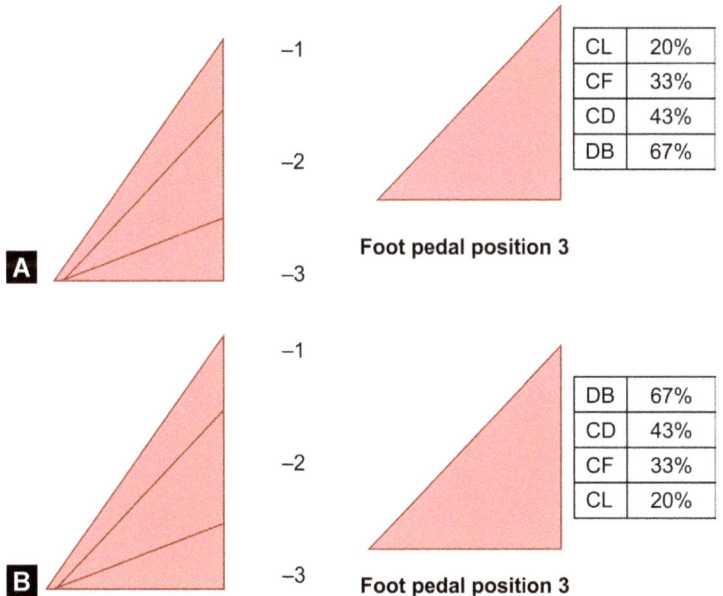

Figs. 11A and B: (A) Variable Whitestar 1; (B) Variable Whitestar 2.

Due to variation in energy mode, it is safe for last pieces also.

The most important advantage is that one can use these variable parameters according to the hardness of nucleus of that particular piece.

Analysis of energy used in Phaco surgery is based on the following points:

Total ultrasound time:
It is the total time during which the ultrasound energy is actually being delivered to emulsify the cataract.

Effective Phaco time:
- It is determined by the Phaco machine; during the surgery, the surgeon uses various percentages of Phaco energy from zero to preset for complete nucleus management (actual Phaco time). Machine denotes that if the surgeon uses its preset values all the time for nucleus management, it will take less duration than needed. This time calculated by the machine is called as effective Phaco time.
- For example, the machine takes 10 seconds with variable percentage of energy to emulsify nucleus; the same mass can be emulsified with continuous preset energy in 3 seconds. So, the actual Phaco time is 10 seconds and effective Phaco time is 3 seconds.

Majority of machines in the market are working with the principle of longitudinal Phaco (traditional Phaco).

COMBINATION OF LONGITUDINAL AND TRANSVERSE FORMS OF ENERGY

Ellips Technology

Principle
- Ellips technology works on the principle of simultaneous longitudinal and transversal delivery of energy (**Fig. 12**).

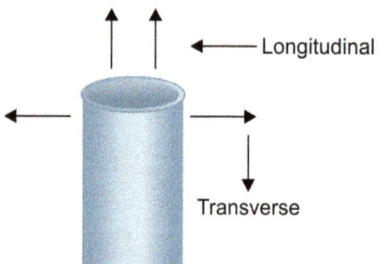

Fig. 12: Ellips technology.

- Longitudinal means to and fro movement and transversal means sideway movement of the Phaco tip.

Advantages
- Better cutting efficiency is due to emulsification of the lens in more than one direction.
- Less repulsion of the nuclear material
- Better followability
- This technology can work with a curved as well as a straight tip.
- During emulsification, clogging of the lens material is less.
- This technology is helpful for hard cataract.

KEY POINTS
- Corneal damage can occur due to energy, so one should have complete knowledge of delivery and different modes of energy used by our own machine.
- One should learn the use of energy with respect to variable density of nucleus.

CHAPTER 4

Vacuum

INTRODUCTION
- This parameter is important for hold and chop and removal of small pieces in nucleus management.
- Vacuum is mainly helpful to hold the nucleus before chop.
- Adequate parameters are set for irrigation aspiration of epinucleus, cortex, and removal of viscoelastic solution.
- Vacuum can be used in panel or linear mode.

PRINCIPLE
- Vacuum means the ability to hold the mass.
- Vacuum transducer is the "Heart" of fluidics pump.

Peristaltic pump:
- When the pump rotates for 4 or 6 notches, fluid is displaced through tubing and negative pressure is created which causes vacuum.
- In a peristaltic pump, negative pressure in the tubing is responsible for hold.
- Vacuum reaches to the preset level, once the tip gets completely occluded.
- If there is a partial occlusion, vacuum will work partially.
- If there is complete occlusion, vacuum will work completely.
- If the Phaco tip occludes nucleus mass with zero-degree effect, one can get complete occlusion (**Fig. 1**).

USES OF VACUUM
- In nucleus management
- For irrigation and aspiration (I/A) of epinucleus and cortex
- Removal of viscoelastic solution, after intraocular lens (IOL) implantation

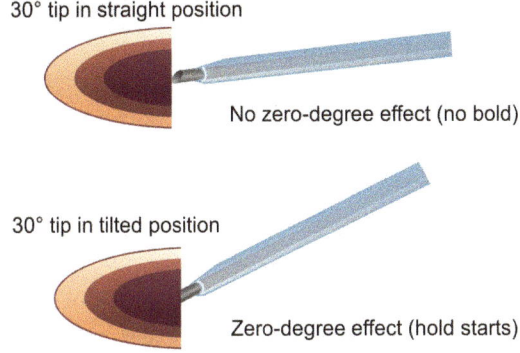

Fig. 1: Mechanism of hold.

DIFFERENT SETTINGS OF VACUUM
Nucleus Management
Trench

In this step, vacuum is needed to remove sculpted nuclear material for better visualization for the next stroke of trench.

Parameters:
- Vacuum can be used as panel or linear.
- 20–50 mm Hg of vacuum can be used.

Trench in different situations:
- *Hard cataract*:
  - Vacuum can be increased >50 mm Hg.
  - It can be kept panel.
- *Soft cataract*:
  - One can decrease the vacuum from 50 to 30 mm Hg.
  - It can be kept linear.
- *Small pupil*:
  - 20–30 mm Hg
  - It can be kept linear.
  - If capsulorhexis is bigger than pupil size, linear vacuum is safe.
- *Shallow anterior chamber*:
  - 20–30 mm Hg
  - Relatively shallow anterior chamber is an important indication for linear vacuum
  - Sometimes, a gap between the anterior capsule and iris is less; try to use linear vacuum.

Some examples:
- *Small pupil with hard cataract*:
  - Vacuum can be linear and kept >50 mm Hg. It means relatively more vacuum but in linear mode.
- *Dilated pupil with hard cataract*:
  - Vacuum can be panel and kept >50 mm Hg. It means relatively more vacuum but in panel mode.

Hold and Consequent Chop

- Vacuum plays the most important role for hold.
- In this step of hold and chop, if your hold is excellent, then chop can occur easily.
- Vacuum in panel mode is generally used for this step.
- Vacuum in linear mode is always safe.

Prerequisite for better hold:
- Adequate mass of nucleus

Principles:
- Angulation of Phaco tip with respect to nucleus mass is the most important factor for better hold.
- It means that zero-degree effect of Phaco tip with respect to nuclear mass is a prerequisite for hold.

Parameters:
- *Normal grade of cataract*:
  - 200–300 mm Hg
  - Vacuum can be used in panel or linear.
- *Hard cataract*:
  - 300–400 mm Hg or more
  - Vacuum can be used in panel.
- *Soft cataract*:
  - 100–200 mm Hg or less
  - Vacuum can be used preferably linear.
- *Small pupil*:
  - 200–250 mm Hg
  - Vacuum can be used linear or panel.
- *Variable anatomy*:
  - In many situations such as deep socket and deep anterior chamber, zero-degree effect is difficult to achieve, where one can increase the vacuum than needed and use panel mode.

Generally, vacuum is used in panel for hold and chop step of nucleus management in stop and chop and direct chop technique.

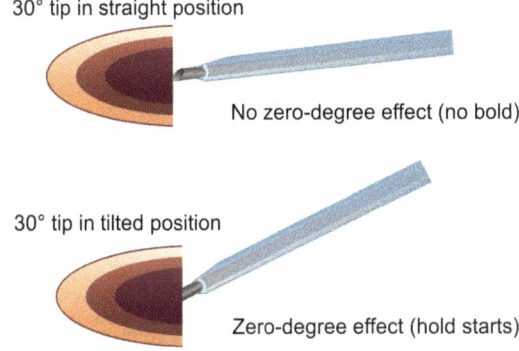

Fig. 1: Mechanism of hold.

DIFFERENT SETTINGS OF VACUUM

Nucleus Management

Trench

In this step, vacuum is needed to remove sculpted nuclear material for better visualization for the next stroke of trench.

Parameters:
- Vacuum can be used as panel or linear.
- 20–50 mm Hg of vacuum can be used.

Trench in different situations:
- *Hard cataract*:
    - Vacuum can be increased >50 mm Hg.
    - It can be kept panel.
- *Soft cataract*:
    - One can decrease the vacuum from 50 to 30 mm Hg.
    - It can be kept linear.
- *Small pupil*:
    - 20–30 mm Hg
    - It can be kept linear.
    - If capsulorhexis is bigger than pupil size, linear vacuum is safe.
- *Shallow anterior chamber*:
    - 20–30 mm Hg
    - Relatively shallow anterior chamber is an important indication for linear vacuum
    - Sometimes, a gap between the anterior capsule and iris is less; try to use linear vacuum.

Some examples:
- *Small pupil with hard cataract*:
  - Vacuum can be linear and kept >50 mm Hg. It means relatively more vacuum but in linear mode.
- *Dilated pupil with hard cataract*:
  - Vacuum can be panel and kept >50 mm Hg. It means relatively more vacuum but in panel mode.

Hold and Consequent Chop

- Vacuum plays the most important role for hold.
- In this step of hold and chop, if your hold is excellent, then chop can occur easily.
- Vacuum in panel mode is generally used for this step.
- Vacuum in linear mode is always safe.

Prerequisite for better hold:
- Adequate mass of nucleus

Principles:
- Angulation of Phaco tip with respect to nucleus mass is the most important factor for better hold.
- It means that zero-degree effect of Phaco tip with respect to nuclear mass is a prerequisite for hold.

Parameters:
- *Normal grade of cataract*:
  - 200–300 mm Hg
  - Vacuum can be used in panel or linear.
- *Hard cataract*:
  - 300–400 mm Hg or more
  - Vacuum can be used in panel.
- *Soft cataract*:
  - 100–200 mm Hg or less
  - Vacuum can be used preferably linear.
- *Small pupil*:
  - 200–250 mm Hg
  - Vacuum can be used linear or panel.
- *Variable anatomy*:
  - In many situations such as deep socket and deep anterior chamber, zero-degree effect is difficult to achieve, where one can increase the vacuum than needed and use panel mode.

Generally, vacuum is used in panel for hold and chop step of nucleus management in stop and chop and direct chop technique.

Common mistakes related to use of vacuum:
- If the surgeon fails to hold the nucleus, generally there is a tendency to increase the vacuum.

Suggestion: Instead of increasing the vacuum suddenly, try to concentrate on achieving zero-degree effect.
- In soft cataract, if the surgeon is unable to hold the mass, there is a tendency to increase the vacuum.

Suggestion: In soft cataract, instead of increasing vacuum, the surgeon should decrease the vacuum for better hold and linear is the better choice than panel.

Removal of Small Pieces

- Among the vacuum and flow rate, flow rate is more important than vacuum.
- Vacuum is having a very specific role for this step.

Role of vacuum:
- Emulsified pieces are aspirated due to vacuum.
- Pieces, which are brought toward Phaco tip, will remain in the vicinity of Phaco tip due to vacuum.
- *Partially occluded tip due to vacuum is the most important prerequisite for better nucleus emulsification.*

Effect of complete and partial occlusion is demonstrated in **Figures 2A and B.**

In complete occlusion, cutting is good but efficiency depends on the location of Phaco tip with respect to nucleus mass.

Due to partial occlusion, Jackhammer effect (to-and-fro movement of Phaco tip) will work more efficiently than complete occlusion.

Formation of air bubbles, which induces cavitational effect, is an important factor for emulsification of nucleus.

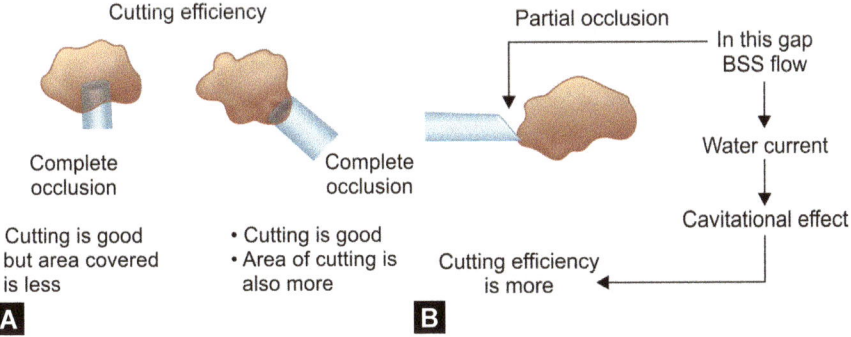

Figs. 2A and B: (A) Effect of complete occlusion; (B) Effect of partial occlusion.

Partial occlusion can be achieved by the following ways:
- Use of 45° Phaco tip
- If surgeon is using 15° or 30° tip which can be applied as a 45° effect
- Vacuum should be adequate, as in high vacuum, tissue can get clogged.
- Pieces can be just repelled away from Phaco tip by gentle touch of chopper.
- In ICE technology, there is a single punch, which will also be helpful to achieve partial occlusion.
- Intelligent Phaco will push the piece away from the Phaco tip to achieve partial occlusion.

Parameters:
- *Normal grade of cataract*:
  - 200–250 mm Hg
  - Vacuum can be kept panel or linear.
- *Hard cataract*:
  - 250–300 mm Hg
  - Vacuum in panel or linear.
- *Soft cataract*:
  - 100–200 mm Hg
  - Vacuum can be kept linear.
- *Shallow anterior chamber*:
  - 150–200 mm Hg
  - Vacuum can be kept linear.
- *Small pupil*:
  - 150–200 mm Hg
  - Vacuum can be kept linear.
- High myopia or deep anterior chamber:
  - 200–300 mm Hg
  - Vacuum can be kept panel/linear.

Irrigation Aspiration of Epinucleus and Cortex

- Irrigation aspiration is for removal of epinucleus and cortex.
- The role of vacuum is important at this step.
- *The surgeon moves cannula to periphery at this step to pull soft tissue, which does not come toward Phaco tip automatically as in the removal of small pieces of nucleus.*

Parameters:
- Generally, vacuum should be kept linear.
- Linear vacuum can be kept from 200 to 400 mm Hg.
- Linear vacuum is safe to avoid catching of iris, capsule, and zonules.
- Surgeon can keep vacuum in panel for better functioning, but parameters should be cut down.

CAP VAC Mode (Polish Mode)

It is used to remove cells or debris from the posterior capsule, polishing and removal of cells from the subcapsular area of anterior capsule and small tags of soft tissue from angle of bag.

Parameters:
- Generally, vacuum should be kept linear.
- Vacuum can be kept from 10 to 14 mm Hg.
- Linear vacuum is safe.
- Vacuum can be kept panel in some cases such as sticky cataract.

Removal of Viscoelastic Solution

- Removal of viscoelastic solution is needed after IOL implantation.
- During this step, an I/A cannula moves 360°.

Parameters
- Vacuum can be kept panel or linear.
- It should be kept little lower than the irrigation aspiration step, i.e., around 100–200 mm Hg.
- Sometimes, removal of viscoelastic solution behind the IOL can be done with low vacuum, i.e., 40–80 mm Hg in linear mode.

DELIVERY SYSTEM OF VACUUM

Vacuum can be used as linear or panel.

Linear Mode

- Gradual increase in the vacuum is called as linear mode.
- It can be preset from lower limit to upper limit.
- Lower limit can start from zero to upper limit up to 500–600 mm Hg.
- Upper limit can be changed according to the anatomy of eye, different grades of cataract, and different types of cataract.

Indication:
- Generally used for normal grades of cataract.
  For example:
  - Grade I-III
  - Shallow anterior chamber
  - Small pupil
  - Soft cataract

Advantages:
- Linear vacuum is safe.
- It is more controlled.

Disadvantage:
Speed of surgery is slow.

Panel Mode
- There is a sudden rise of vacuum to preset level (related to occlusion).
- Panel vacuum can be set up to 200–500 mm Hg as a higher limit.

Indication:
- Generally used for the harder nucleus
  For example:
  - If it is more than grade IV, panel vacuum can be used safely.
  - High myopia

Advantages:
- Control on hold of nucleus mass is more.
- Duration of hold is more as compared to linear.
- Speed of surgery is fast.

Disadvantages:
- Less surgical control with panel vacuum
- Chances of catching iris during nucleus management
- Chances of catching anterior capsule, posterior capsule, iris when bag is empty that is during I/A of epinucleus and cortex

KEY POINTS

To achieve good vacuum:
- Use of adequate parameters mainly for hold of the nucleus
- Angulation of Phaco tip with respect to nuclear mass is important.
- Zero-degree effect between Phaco tip with nucleus
- Change of parameters of vacuum related to density of nucleus

Adequate vacuum is not only important to hold but also to maintain the hold of nucleus for better chopping.

CHAPTER 5

Aspiration Flow Rate

INTRODUCTION
- This parameter is important for hold and chop and removal of small pieces in nucleus management.
- Flow rate is mainly helpful in quadrant removal.
- Adequate parameters are set for irrigation and aspiration of epinucleus, cortex, and removal of viscoelastic solution.
- Balance between irrigation flow and aspiration flow rate is important to avoid surge.
- Flow rate can be used in linear or panel mode.

PRINCIPLE
- Amount of fluid coming out of the eye in cc/min
- Ability of followability of the tissue is due to flow rate (**Fig. 1**).

USES
- In nucleus management
- In irrigation and aspiration of epinucleus and cortex
- In removal of viscoelastic after intraocular lens (IOL) implantation

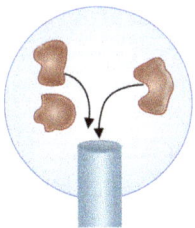

Movement of pieces toward the Phaco tip is due to flow rate

Fig. 1: Principle of flow rate.

DIFFERENT SETTINGS OF FLOW RATE

Nucleus Management

Trench

In this step, flow rate is needed to aspirate the emulsified material.

Parameters:
- Adequate flow rate 10–20 cc/min.
- It can be panel or linear.

Hold and Chop

- Role of flow rate is to bring the nucleus and to maintain the vicinity of nucleus related to Phaco tip.
- Parameters can be increased or decreased according to density of the nucleus.
- Delivery mode can be panel or linear according to the density of the nucleus.
- Parameters and delivery mode vary according to location of hold of nucleus.

Parameters:
- *For normal grade of cataract*:
  - Flow rate is 24–30 cc/min.
  - Flow rate can be kept panel or linear.
- *Hard cataract*:
  - Flow rate is 30–36 cc/min.
  - Flow rate can be kept panel.
- *Soft cataract*:
  - Flow rate is 20–24 cc/min.
  - Linear flow rate is for better control.
- Many times, the surgeon has to hold the nucleus away from the center, i.e., in the periphery to lift it out of the bag:
  - Cut down the parameters of flow rate from 24 to 20 cc/min.
  - Delivery of flow rate shifted from panel to linear.

Removal of Small Pieces of Nucleus (Quadrant Removal) (Figs. 2A and B)

- Flow rate is one of the most important and crucial factors in the removal of small pieces of nucleus.
- Pieces come toward the Phaco tip due to the flow rate.
- Many other factors such as number of incisions and number of instruments passing in anterior chamber are responsible for good flow rate.

Aspiration Flow Rate

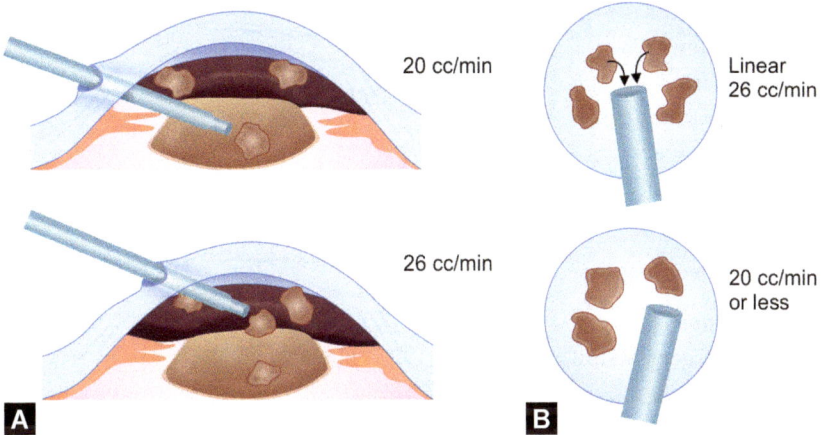

Figs. 2A and B: (A) Anteroposterior position of Phaco tip in quadrant removal; (B) Horizontal position of Phaco tip in quadrant removal.

Parameters:
- Flow rate is 24–28 cc/min.
- Delivery mode is generally linear for safety and panel for fast procedure.

Parameters of flow rate do not really depend on the hardness of nucleus but these depend on anatomy of eyeball.

Delivery System of Flow Rate

Flow rate can be used as linear or panel.

Linear Mode

- Gradual increase in the flow rate is called linear flow rate.
- It can be preset from lower limit to upper limit.
- Lower limit can start from zero to upper limit up to 40 cc/min.
- Upper limit can be changed according to the anatomy of eye, different grades of cataract, and different types of cataract.
- In quadrant removal, multiple pieces are wandering in the anterior chamber and bag. In such a situation when Phaco tip is near the center, the surgeon can use higher parameters which are preset and can be decreased when the Phaco tip is moving away from center (horizontally or anteroposteriorly) which is possible in linear mode (**Figs. 2A** and **B**).

Indications:
- Shallow anterior chamber
- Small pupil
- Shallow bag

- Small eye
- Hypermetropia
- Floppy iris
- Positive pressure
- Hazy cornea
- When capsulorhexis is bigger than iris

Advantage:
Linear mode is safe.

Disadvantage:
Speed of surgery is slow.

Panel Mode
- Flow rate will reach to preset level suddenly once foot pedal is pressed.
- Using panel mode for this step needs more experience.
- Parameters should be adequate.

Indications:
- Normal anatomy
- Deep anterior chamber
- Well-dilated pupil
- Deep bag
- Myopia
- Hard cataract
- Cortical and sticky cataract
- In cases of posterior capsule rupture (PCR)
- After anterior vitrectomy

Advantages:
Procedure will be fast. Procedure should be fast in some situations such as:
- When patient is not comfortable.
- In PCR, when pieces are wandering in anterior chamber.
- In hard cataract with multiple pieces, the panel mode is a good option for removal of pieces fast to avoid corneal damage.

Disadvantages:
- Less surgical control
- Chances of catching iris, capsule, and sometimes Descemet's membrane are quite common.

Irrigation and Aspiration of Epinucleus and Cortex
- This step is always in an empty bag.
- Epinucleus and cortex are situated near iris, anterior, and posterior capsule.

Parameters:
- Flow rate is 15–20 cc/min
- Delivery mode is generally linear or panel.
- For sticky and thick epinucleus, the panel mode is better option.

CAP-VAC Mode

In this step, debris or cells have to be removed from posterior capsule, beneath the anterior capsule and at the junction of anterior and posterior capsules.

Parameters
- Flow rate is 5–10 cc/min.
- Delivery mode is generally linear.

Removal of Viscoelastic Solution

- Viscoelastic removal is an important step to avoid postoperative inflammation and raised intraocular pressure.
- Removal of viscoelastic is from the anterior chamber, capsular bag, and anterior and posterior aspect of IOL.

Parameters:
Parameters are nearly the same as in cortex removal or they can be reduced.
- Flow rate is 12–18 cc/min.
- Delivery mode is generally linear; sometimes, it may be panel.

Sometimes, one has to remove viscoelastic behind the IOL or from the periphery; at that time, one can cut down the parameters.
- Flow rate is 10–14 cc/min.
- Linear mode is safe.

KEY POINTS

How to achieve good flow rate:
- Use of adequate parameters mainly for quadrant removal step
- Less number of incisions
- Number of instruments used in the anterior chamber should be less.
- Number of times instruments entered in the anterior chamber should be as minimal as possible.
- Pressure of Phaco probe and chopper on incision site is important to avoid leakage which in turn affects aspiration flow rate.
- Architecture of the incisions (main and side port) is crucial point.
- Horizontal water current of irrigation flow is an important factor, which assists the flow rate.

CHAPTER 6

Association of Energy Vacuum and Flow Rate

INTRODUCTION

- Understanding the association of energy, vacuum, and flow rate with each other is the most important factor for a better surgical outcome.
- In peristaltic pump, flow rate and vacuum work independently but assist each other.
- Customizing the parameters of vacuum, flow rate, and energy depends on case to case and surgeon to surgeon.
- Mismatch in use of these parameters can cause surge.

IMPORTANT FACTORS RELATED TO ASSOCIATION OF ENERGY, VACUUM, AND FLOW RATE

- Occlusion mode
- Ice technology
- Intelligent Phaco (IP)
- Surge

Occlusion Mode

- In occlusion mode, one can set preocclusion and postocclusion parameters of vacuum and flow rate. One can also change energy modulation in pre- and postocclusion stages.
- In this mode, there is association of vacuum, flow rate, and energy to each other in preocclusion and postocclusion steps of nucleus management.
- Mainly correlation of vacuum and flow rate is to maintain the anterior chamber stability.
- It is a two-line setting and used for hold and chop and removal of small pieces.
- This mode is important to avoid surge.
- When foot pedal is pressed, flow rate will reach to 30 cc/min.
    - At this point, vacuum reaches to 100 mm Hg, which sends the machine in *preocclusion stage*.

Association of Energy Vacuum and Flow Rate

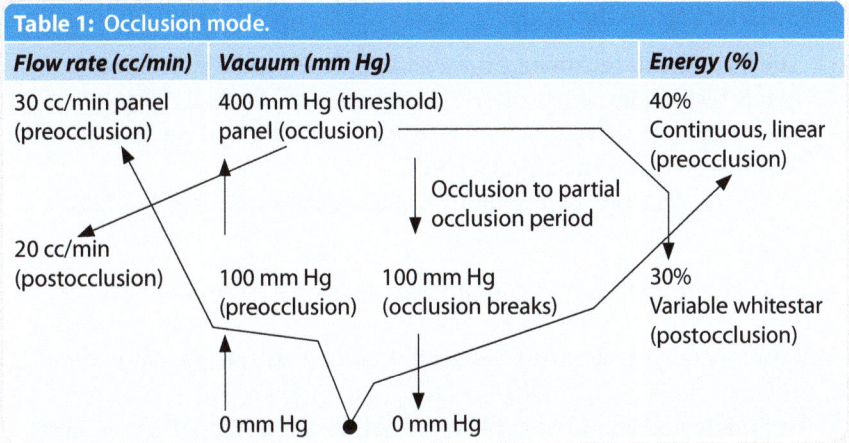

Table 1: Occlusion mode.

- Once vacuum built from 100 to 400 mm Hg, the machine starts working in *occlusion stage*.
  At this stage, flow rate will drop down to 20 cc/min.
  - When occlusion breaks, i.e., *postocclusion stage*, vacuum drops down from 400 to 100 mm Hg but aspiration flow rate is maintained to 20 cc/min.

  This will avoid chances of sudden gush of fluid inside the tubing which can cause instability of anterior chamber.

  When vacuum drops from 100 to 0 mm Hg, it again works at a preocclusion stage of 30 cc/min and new cycle starts.

In normal physics:
- *Flow rate*: Once the piece is occluded, flow rate will go from 30 to 0 cc/min.
- *Vacuum*: When tip is occluded completely, vacuum works at 400 mm Hg. With sudden occlusion break, vacuum will go to 0 mm Hg.

In this occlusion mode:
- Role of flow rate in the following occlusion stages:
  - *Preocclusion stage*: Higher flow rate for better followability
  - *Postocclusion stage*: Lower flow rate for better safety
- Aspiration flow rate of 20 cc/min and 100 mm Hg vacuum is a speed breaker for safety (which maintains the anterior chamber to avoid "surge").

ICE Technology

Increased controlled and efficiency:
- Pulse-shaping technology
- Case technology

Pulse-shaping Technology

- The form of this technology is ascending, fixed, and descending.
- In this technology, one can get 1 ms additional punch.
- This punch gives a space between Phaco needle and nuclear material, which accelerates cavitational effect.
- This additional punch amplitude can be customized from 1 to 12%.

Principles:

Punch mechanically pushes nuclear material away from Phaco tip.
↓
Allow creation of microvoid between occluded tip and nuclear material.
↓
This microvoid allows fresh balanced salt solution (BSS) to create fresh bubbles and creation of cavitational effect.
↓
Fresh BSS interacts with ultrasound power to accelerate cavitational effect, by forming new air bubble.
↓
Hence, it increases efficiency of ultrasound power.
↓

Advantages:

- Mainly used for the removal of small pieces.
- This additional punch will redirect the pieces, which is really helpful.
- Effective Phaco time is reduced.
- This can be superimposed on other form of power modulations such as:
  - Short pulse
  - Long pulse
  - Burst mode
  - Low power pulse
  - High power pulse
  - Continuous mode

Case Technology

Chamber stabilization environment:

- This is based on working zone and safety zone.
- Four parameters can be preset:
  - Case vacuum
  - Up threshold
  - Down threshold
  - Up time

1. *Case vacuum*:
   - If a surgeon is comfortable with 300 mm Hg vacuum, then one can set the desired vacuum of 400–450 mm Hg (in hard cataract) but will get safety of 300 mm Hg (comfortable vacuum).

2. *Up time:*
   - It decides how much time to work with high vacuum (preset, e.g., 450 mm Hg)
   - This can be customized to 200–2,000 ms.
   - It indicates the time, where the surgeon can be at higher vacuum (performing time) for that period.
3. *Down threshold:*
   - 150–170 mm Hg which is preset and recovers once the fall-down of vacuum from 300 not to 0 but to preset. So, it regains faster and starts a new cycle.
   - It is a parameter which can be set for reachieving the desired occlusion.
   - If one has set down threshold 150 mm Hg. At occlusion break, generally vacuum breaks down to 0, but the machine will immediately sense the preset vacuum within 26 ms.
4. *Up threshold:*
   - It is 95% of preset vacuum.
   - It is the sensor of machine to start the timer.

Fusion fluidics is the combination of case mode and occlusion mode.

Intelligent Phaco

- Intelligent Phaco is a feature used in torsional technology in quadrant removal step.
- In foot pedal position 3, when Phaco tip clogged nuclear material at a threshold of 85–90% of preset vacuum, IP starts and pushes the nuclear material and keeps it at an ideal plane for use of shearing forces for emulsification.

Advantages

- It enhances emulsification of the nucleus and thus improves efficiency.
- Preset vacuum is not achieved so the pump keeps on turning which improves the followability of the nucleus material toward tip
- Decreases intraocular pressure fluctuation which in turn reduces surge during surgery
- Decreases use of energy into the eye

Surge

- This is the most important happening during Phaco surgery.
- Collapse of anterior chamber due to sudden gush of fluid from the anterior chamber to the aspiration port of the Phaco tip or I/A cannula, once the occlusion break is called surge
- Surge occurs mainly during hold and chop, removal of pieces, and sometimes during irrigation and aspiration (I/A) step

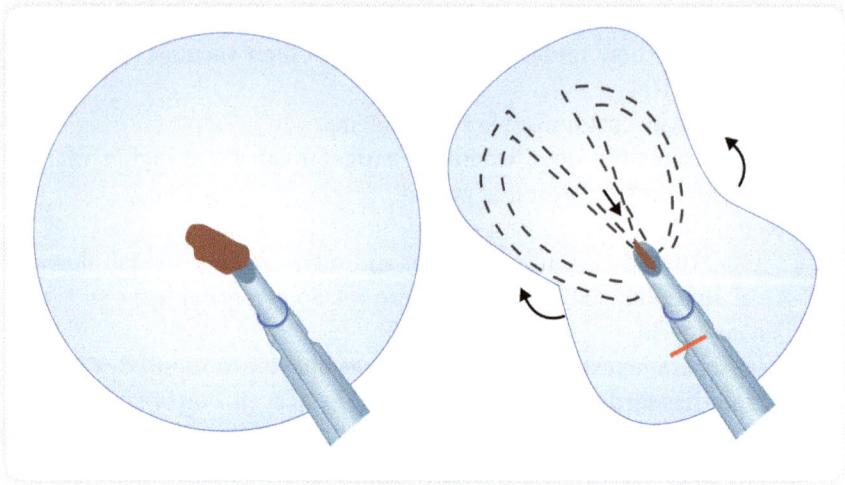

Fig. 1: Mechanism of surge.

- Surge occurs due to lack of knowledge about how to use parameters of vacuum and flow rate in association with each other.

During the removal of nucleus pieces, when the piece is away from the Phaco tip, the rollers rotate and no occlusion or collapse of tubing occurs, but when the Phaco tip gets occluded, vacuum builds up, pump stops, and a negative pressure is generated within the system and tubing gets collapsed. After break of occlusion at one point, pressure is released and the tubing expands to the original size and fluid is drawn from the anterior chamber to fill up this extra-volume of the tubing and the anterior chamber can get collapsed (**Fig. 1**).

Factors Responsible for Surge

- If vacuum and flow rate are in panel
- Mismatch between parameters of flow rate and vacuum
- Among the vacuum and flow rate parameters, the flow rate is responsible factor for surge
- If the quality of the tubing is not good
- If irrigation flow is less
- Improper architecture of incisions
- Wound leakage
- Control of foot pedal

Complications due to Surge

- Posterior capsule rupture
- Iris trauma
- Endothelial damage

How to Avoid Surge?

- Increase the infusion fluid by:
  - Increasing the bottle height
  - Using the transurethral resection (TUR) set or wide-bore intravenous (IV) cannula
  - Additional infusion by anterior chamber maintainer
  - Use of air pump to increase the flow
- *Parameters*:
  - Decrease the parameters of aspiration flow rate and vacuum
  - Vacuum and flow rate can be shifted from panel to linear.
  - Correlation of flow rate and vacuum will work together to decrease the surge.
  - Basically, aspiration flow rate is having an important role to avoid surge.
- *Incision*:
  - Avoid leakage from incision which is an important factor for surge:
    - Proper wound construction of main and side port
    - Avoid pressure of Phaco tip and chopper on incision during surgery
- *Foot pedal*:
  - Foot pedal control is one of the most important aspects to avoid surge.
  - To move from foot pedal position II to III and back from III to II, one should be very well coordinated with step of surgery, i.e., chopping or emulsifying of nucleus pieces.
- *During surgery*:
  - During the removal of small pieces or I/A of epinucleus and cortex, the Phaco tip or I/A port should be in opposition with the next mass before occlusion breaks.
- *Machine*:
  - Some machines have sensor which detects occlusion break and avoids surge by release of fluid or air into the system.
  - New software in the machine such as occlusion mode and case mode is important to avoid surge.
  - Disposable tubings are better to avoid surge.

KEY POINTS

- Association of energy, vacuum, and flow rate plays a vital role in completion of Phaco surgery in a better way.
- Knowledge of definition, principle, delivery mode, parameters related to energy, vacuum and flow rate, and their correlation with each other is important to use the Phaco machine with its better efficiency.
- New software in the machines is developed on the basis of these principles.

CHAPTER 7

Torsional Technology

INTRODUCTION

- Torsional technology is called Ozil technology.
- Kelman tip is used.
- Angulation of tip is 45°.
- Mini flared tip with bore size 0.9 mm is commonly used.
- Disposable cassette is used for prime and tuning of the machine.
- This is incorporated in Alcon machine.

PRINCIPLE

- Use of oscillatory torsional amplitude at the tip end to facilitate a lateral tip movement from one side to the other side
- Tip oscillates 32,000 times per second (32,000 Hz) from side to side.
- Oscillations are 3.6 mil of stroke at cutting edge and 1.6 mil at incision site.

Cutting of tissue is by shearing forces.

ADVANTAGES

- Due to Kelman tip, surgeon can get all the advantages of the curved tip.
- Cutting efficiency is excellent due to:
  - Torsional technology (**Fig. 1**)
  - 45° angulation of tip

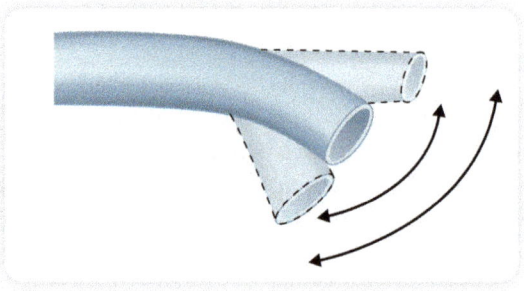

Fig. 1: Torsional technology.

- Combination of longitudinal as well as torsional energy can be possible simultaneously
- Less repulsion of nuclear pieces which improves followability
- Duration for emulsification is less.
- Heat generation is less.
- Corneal burn is less.
- Use of disposable cassette is mandatory:
  - Chance of infection is less.
  - Flow of irrigating fluid is excellent.
  - Efficiency of vacuum and flow rate is good.
- This machine is efficient in removal of hard cataract.

MACHINE FEATURES

Irrigation

- Bottle height is 110 cm, which can be decreased up to 35 or 13 cm.
- Automatically adjustable irrigating stand
- Machine uses custom fluidics software based on gravity flow.

CDE Metrics

- It is the cumulative dissipated energy.
- It is a very important evaluator point.
- It is designed to monitor the amount of energy delivered during phacoemulsification.

This unique feature will give an idea about:
- *Ultrasound*:
  - Total time
  - Total equivalent power in position 3
  - Cumulative dissipated energy
- *Phaco time*:
  - Average Phaco power
  - Average Phaco power in position 3
- *Torsional amplitude*:
  - It is the maximum distance moved by a point and vibrating body or wave measured from its equilibrium position
  - Torsional time
  - Average torsional amplitude
  - Average torsional amplitude in position 3
  - Equivalent torsional amplitude in position 3
- *Neosonics*:
  - Oscillations controlled independent of ultrasound
  - Neosonics time
  - Average neosonics power

- *Fluidics:*
    - Aspiration time
    - Estimated fluid used
- *Aqua Lase:*
    - It uses the balanced salt solution (BSS) pulses to dissolve the lens.
    - Aqua Lase time
    - Aqua Lase number of pulses
    - Average Aqua Lase magnitude
    - Average Aqua Lase magnitude in position 3

Foot Pedal

It is an enhanced foot switch:
- Buttons
- Treadle
- Vibration (On or Off)
- Detent firmness
- Span

Span for position zero is 5%.
  General position for span is as shown in **Figure 2**.
- Spans 2 and 3 are very significant
- Hold and chop is better, if span 2 is adequate.
- Cutting starts suddenly, if span 3 is more.

Energy

- Ozil technology is a torsional technology.
- Cutting is by shearing forces.
- Cutting efficiency is more by placing Phaco tip just near to piece.
- Ozil can be used as:
    - Ozil continuous
    - Ozil pulse
    - Ozil burst

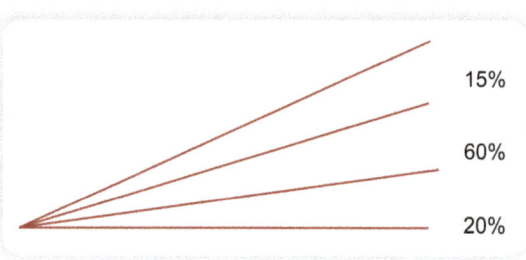

Fig. 2: General position for span.

Ozil Continuous

- Torsional amplitude in percentage:
  - Limits from 0 to 100
  - Can be linear or panel
- Phaco power:
  - *Limits*: Upper and lower
  - Can be linear as well as panel

Features of Ozil continuous:
- Phaco power
- Torsional amplitude
- Vacuum
- Aspiration flow rate

Uses of Ozil continuous:
- Trench
- For removal of small pieces
- Sometimes to remove epinucleus
- It is usually linear
- Foot pedal control is most important in Ozil continuous.

Ozil Pulse

- Works on the basis of on and off time
- Torsional amplitude works in pulse also
- One can set lower and upper limits
- On and off time can be modified

Ozil Burst

- Energy used in panel mode is called burst mode.
- Torsional amplitude is also working which can be set from lower to upper limit.
- On time and off time can be set.

For example:
- On time = 50 ms, off time = 50 ms, power = 30, and torsional amplitude = 0
- One can increase on time and off time up to 500 ms.
- Initially, there is an off time of 500 ms. As you press the foot pedal more and more, it decreases gradually every time by 50 and when you press the foot pedal and reach to the end, then one can get 50 ms on time and 50 ms off time.

Dynamic Rise

It is temporarily used to increase or decrease the flow rate as per requirement during hold and chop and removal of nucleus pieces.

For example:
- In dynamic rise +1, during the time of occlusion, the flow rate increases by 25% temporarily; in this period, the rotation of pump also increases to build up the required vacuum in less time.
- In dynamic rise −1, during the time of occlusion, the flow rate decreases by 25%.

SURGICAL PARAMETERS

Sculpt

Energy:
- Phaco power: 0
- Ozil continuous in linear
- Torsional amplitude: 0-100%.
- Dynamic rise: 0

Vacuum:
- 30-50 mm Hg in panel

Aspiration flow rate:
- 20-30 cc/min in panel

Use:
- All grades of cataract

Variation:
- In hard cataract, one can use Phaco power from 40 to 70% along with torsional in linear mode
- In soft cataract:
  - Torsional amplitude can be used from 0 to 70%.
  - Sometimes, one can use Phaco power from 50 to 60% only without torsional mode.

Custom 1

Energy:
- *Phaco power*: 30-50% linear
- *Torsional amplitude*: 0

Vacuum:
- 300-400 mm Hg in panel

Aspiration flow rate:
- 30-40 cc/min in panel

Use:
- For hold and chop of nucleus in hard cataract

Variation:
- In very hard cataract (more than grades V and VI), these parameters can be still increased.

Quadrant Removal

Energy:
- Phaco power: 0
- Torsional amplitude: 0–100%
- *Intelligent Phaco (IP) is on.*

When IP is set at 90% of vacuum, it means that in foot position 3, once the vacuum reaches to 90% of preset vacuum, it pushes and redirects the pieces of nucleus to keep it away from the Phaco tip and at the plane of shearing forces for better cutting efficiency.

Vacuum:
- 250–350 mm Hg in panel

Aspiration flow rate:
- 30–35 cc/min in pancl or linear

Use:
- For removal of small pieces of nucleus

Variation:
- In hard cataract:
  - Phaco power can be used 20–30% along with torsional mode.
  - Vacuum and aspiration flow rate can be increased and used in panel mode.
- In soft cataract:
  - Ozil pulse can be used.
  - Vacuum and flow rate can be decreased and used in linear mode.
  - Sometimes, vacuum can be used in panel and flow rate in linear mode.

Chop

Energy:
- Phaco power: 20–40%
- Torsional amplitude: 0

Vacuum:
- 200–300 mm Hg in panel

Aspiration flow rate:
- 20–30 cc/min in panel

Use:
- For hold and chop of nucleus in grades II and III cataract

Variation:
- In hard cataract, parameters can be increased.
- In soft cataract, parameters can be decreased.

Custom 2

Energy:
- Phaco power: 10–20%, linear
- Torsional amplitude: 0

Vacuum:
- 120–180 mm Hg and can be panel/linear.

Aspiration flow rate:
- 14–24 cc/min and can be linear/panel

Uses:
- For hold and lift of nucleus in soft cataract
- For hold and lift of epinucleus mainly in sticky cataract

Variation:
- In very soft cataracts, parameters can be still reduced.

Epinucleus Mode

Energy:
- Phaco power: 0
- Torsional amplitude: Can be kept from 0 to 50% linear

Vacuum:
- 120–160 mm Hg and can be panel/linear

Aspiration flow rate:
- 10–24 cc/min and can be linear/panel

Uses:
- For removal of epinucleus
- Can be used for removal of the last small pieces of nucleus
- In very soft cataract, for nucleus and epinucleus removal

Cortex

Vacuum:
- 300–400 mm Hg and linear/panel

Aspiration flow rate:
- 20–30 cc/min and linear/panel

Uses:
- For removal of cortex
- For removal of epinuclear sheet
- For removal of viscoelastic

Variation:
- Both the vacuum and flow rate can be used either linear or panel according to the anatomical variation.

For example:
Generally, parameters are in linear mode but can be used in panel mode for sticky and thick epinucleus.
- If parameters are used in panel, they can be decreased.
- Parameters can be decreased while going near the weak zone.

Polish

Vacuum:
- 5-10 mm Hg and linear

Aspiration flow rate:
- 5-10 cc/min and linear

Uses:
- For polishing of cells over the posterior capsule and subcapsular epithelial cells of the anterior capsule
- For removal of small strands of cortical fibers from the posterior capsule, posterior aspect of the anterior capsule, and junction between both the capsules

Variation:
- After catching cortical fibers in polish mode from periphery, if bulk is big, then shift from polish to cortex mode is important.

Viscoelastic Removal

Vacuum:
- 120-160 mm Hg and panel/linear

Aspiration flow rate:
- 10-24 cc/min and linear/panel

Use:
- For removal of viscoelastic after IOL implantation

Variation:
- Vacuum and flow rate are used in panel in the center and linear at periphery.

- Parameters used in linear are important for removal of viscoelastic from behind the IOL and over the posterior capsule.
- If parameters are used in panel, it should be decreased for safety.

Anterior Vitrectomy

Cutting:
- 600–2,500 CPM (cutting per minute)

Vacuum:
- 200–250 mm Hg and can be panel/linear.

Aspiration flow rate:
- 20–28 cc/min and can be linear/panel.
- Bottle height can be reduced.

Uses:
- For anterior and mid vitrectomy

Variation:
- Parameter varies according to different situations, which occurs after PCR.
- After anterior vitrectomy, one can change parameter to irrigation and aspiration (I/A) mode to remove the epinucleus or cortical fibers from periphery.

DISADVANTAGES

- Showering of the lens material
- Learning curve is more due to use of Kelman tip
- It is difficult to understand plane of nucleus with respect to the distal end of Phaco tip.

CENTURION VISION SYSTEM

Principle
- It works on the principle of torsional Phaco with new software.
- This system incorporates active fluidics, which maintains excellent chamber and pressure stability.
- Use of intrepid balanced tip and infusion sleeve with its unique design giving advantage of more torsional movement at the distal end of tip and at the same time less tip movement at incision site.

Advantages
- All the advantages of torsional technology
- Excellent chamber stability

- Maintain natural intraocular pressure of the eye
- Due to customization of the intraocular pressure, this machine is helpful for cataract associated with conditions such as myopia, hypotony, weak zonules, and post-vitrectomized eyes.

KEY POINTS

- Surgeons started getting knowledge and advantage of angulated tip.
- This different technology is very helpful for hard cataract removal.

CHAPTER 8

Phaco Parameters in Different Types of Cataract

INTRODUCTION

- Setting of parameters in the Phaco machine is one of the crucial factors for successful Phaco surgery.
- One should know the definition and meaning of vacuum, flow rate, and energy.
- Understanding the association of vacuum, flow rate, and energy is important.
- It needs time to understand this combination of parameters.
- Sometimes, parameters differ machine to machine and surgeon to surgeon.
- With experience, one can customize this combination of parameters in a better way.
- Working of parameters is based on control of foot pedal.
- Use of linear or panel delivery system for vacuum and flow rate is really an art to be learned by everyone.

MODES

- Energy:
  - Generally used in linear mode
- Vacuum:
  - Mainly used in panel and sometimes linear in nucleus management
  - Generally kept in linear for irrigation and aspiration of epinucleus and cortex
- Flow rate:
  - Mainly used in panel during hold and chop step of nucleus management
  - Generally used in linear during quadrant removal step of nucleus management
  - Used in linear mode for irrigation-aspiration of epinucleus and cortex

Delivery system of vacuum and flow rate:
- Linear
- Panel

Advantages

Linear mode:
- Procedure is controlled.
- It is generally safe.

Panel mode:
- Procedure is fast.
- It works like a venturi pump.

PARAMETERS IN THE FORM OF CHART

E: Energy, V: Vacuum, FR: Flow rate
  Normal cataract means grades III and IV density of nucleus.

Longitudinal (Traditional) Phaco

Most of the machines are based on the principle of longitudinal Phaco.
- Normal cataract
- Hard cataract
- Soft cataract
- Mature cataract
- Normal cataract in myopia/deep anterior chamber
- Normal cataract in shallow anterior chamber/hypermetropia
- Cataract with pseudoexfoliation (normal grade)
- Very hard cataract with normal anatomy
- Cataract with hazy cornea or corneal opacity
- Cataract with mid dilated pupil
- Diffuse or sticky cataract (normal grade)
- Cortical cataract (normal grade)
- Diabetic cataract
- Normal cataract with floppy iris
- Hard cataract with floppy iris
- Cataract with vitreous opacity (normal grade)

Phaco Parameters in Different Types of Cataract

1. *Normal cataract:*

	E (%)	V (mm Hg)	FR (cc/min)	Remarks
Trench	60–70 Continuous Linear	20–40 Panel/Linear	10–20 Panel/Linear	
Hold and chop	a. 20–40 Continuous Linear	250–300 Linear	26–32 Linear	Safe, controlled
	b. 20–40 Continuous Linear	250–300 Panel	26–32 Panel	Fast, strong
	c. 20–40 Continuous Linear	250–300 Panel	26–32 Linear	Safe, fast, and controlled
Removal of pieces	a. 20–30 Linear Hyperpulse/ Pulse	200–250 Panel/Linear	26–30 Linear	Safe, controlled
	b. 20–30 Linear Hyperpulse/ Pulse	200–250 Panel/Linear	26–30 Panel	Fast

2. *Hard cataract:*

	E (%)	V (mm Hg)	FR (cc/min)	Remarks
Trench	70–80 Continuous Linear	30–50 Panel/Linear	20–26 Panel/Linear	Sharp or new tip is recommended
Hold and chop	30–50 Continuous Linear	300–400 Panel	26–36 Panel	
Removal of pieces	a. 30–40 Linear Hyperpulse/ Pulse/ Long pulse	250–300 Panel	26–34 Linear	Safe and controlled
	b. 30–40 Linear Hyperpulse/ Pulse/ Long pulse	250–300 Panel	26–34 Panel	Fast

3. *Soft cataract*:

	E (%)	V (mm Hg)	FR (cc/min)	Remarks
Trench	50–60 Continuous Linear	20–40 Panel/Linear	10–20 Linear/Panel	Speed of trench should be fast
Hold and chop	20–30 or Sometime <20 Continuous Linear Hyperpulse/Pulse	100–200 Linear/Panel	20–26 Linear/Panel	This step should be done slowly
Removal of pieces	20–30 Linear Hyperpulse/ Pulse/Short pulse	100–200 Panel/Linear	20–26 Linear/Panel Or 20–24 Panel	

4. *Mature cataract*:

	E (%)	V (mm Hg)	FR (cc/min)	Remarks
Trench	60–70 Continuous Linear	20–40 Panel/Linear	10–20 Panel/Linear	
Hold and chop	20–30 Continuous Linear	250–300 Panel/Linear	22–30 Panel/Linear	Energy, vacuum and flow rate according to density of nucleus
Removal of pieces	20–30 Linear Hyperpulse/Pulse	200–250 Linear/Panel	24–28 Linear/Panel	

5. *Normal cataract in myopia/deep anterior chamber*:

	E (%)	V (mm Hg)	FR (cc/min)	Remarks
Trench	60–70 Continuous Linear	20–40 Panel/Linear	10–20 Panel/Linear	
Hold and chop	20–30 Continuous Linear	200–350 Panel/Linear	26–34 Panel/Linear	
Removal of pieces	20–30 Linear Hyperpulse/ Pulse	200–300 Panel/Linear	24–30 Panel/Linear	Parameters are in panel as working space is more

6. *Normal cataract in shallow anterior chamber/hypermetropia:*

	E (%)	V (mm Hg)	FR (cc/min)	Remarks
Trench	60–70 or less Continuous Linear	20–40 Panel/Linear	10–20 Linear/Panel	
Hold and chop	20–30 Continuous Linear	200–250 Panel/Linear	24–28 Panel/Linear	
Removal of pieces	20–30 Linear Hyperpulse/Pulse	150–200 Panel/Linear	20–26 Linear/Panel	Linear is safe

7. *Cataract with pseudoexfoliation (normal grade):*

	E (%)	V (mm Hg)	FR (cc/min)	Remarks
Trench	60–70 Continuous Linear	20–40 Panel/Linear	10–20 Panel/Linear	Energy according to density of nucleus to avoid pressure on zonules
Hold and chop	20–30 Continuous Linear	250–300 Panel/Linear	20–30 Panel/Linear	
Removal of pieces	20–30 Linear Hyperpulse/Pulse	200–250 Panel/Linear	24–28 Linear/Panel	

8. *Very hard cataract with normal anatomy*:

	E (%)	V (mm Hg)	FR (cc/min)	Remarks
Trench	70–80 Continuous Linear/Burst mode	20–50 Panel/Linear	20–28 Panel/Linear	Sharp tip is recommended
Hold and chop	30–50 Continuous Linear	300–400 or 450 Panel/Linear	30–40 Panel/Linear	
Removal of pieces	30–40 Linear Hyperpulse	250–350 Panel/Linear	30–36 Panel/Linear	Due to panel, procedure can be fast

Phaco Parameters in Different Types of Cataract

9. *Cataract with hazy cornea or corneal opacity*:

	E (%)	V (mm Hg)	FR (cc/min)	Remarks
Trench	60–70 Continuous Linear	20–40 Panel/Linear	10–20 Panel/Linear	
Hold and chop	20–30 Continuous Linear	200–300 Panel/Linear	24–30 Panel/Linear	
Removal of pieces	20–30 Linear Hyperpulse/Pulse/Short pulse	200–250 Panel/Linear	24–28 Linear/Panel	Dispersive viscoelastic for protection of endothelium

10. *Cataract in mid-dilated pupil*:

	E (%)	V (mm Hg)	FR (cc/min)	Remarks
Trench	60–70 or less Continuous Linear	20–40 Linear/Panel	10–20 Linear/Panel	
Hold and chop	20–30 Continuous Linear	200–250 Panel/Linear	24–28 Linear/Panel	
Removal of pieces	20–30 Linear Hyperpulse/ Pulse/Short pulse	150–200 Linear/Panel	20–24 Linear/Panel	Linear mode is safe to avoid catching of iris

11. *Diffuse or sticky cataract (normal grade)*:

	E (%)	V (mm Hg)	FR (cc/min)	Remarks
Trench	60–70 Continuous Linear	20–40 Panel/Linear	10–20 Panel/Linear	
Hold and chop	20–30 Continuous Linear	200–300 Panel/Linear	26–30 Panel/Linear	
Removal of pieces	20–30 Linear Hyperpulse/ Pulse/Short pulse/Long pulse	200–250 Panel/Linear	20–28 Panel/Linear	

12. *Cortical cataract (normal grade)*:

	E (%)	V (mm Hg)	FR (cc/min)	Remarks
Trench	60–70 Continuous Linear	20–40 Panel/Linear	10–20 Panel/Linear	
Hold and chop	20–30 Continuous Linear	200–300 Panel/Linear	20–30 Panel/Linear	This step should be done slowly
Removal of pieces	20–30 Linear Hyperpulse/Pulse	200–250 Panel/Linear	22–28 Panel/Linear	

13. *Diabetic cataract*:

	E (%)	V (mm Hg)	FR (cc/min)	Remarks
Trench	60–70 Continuous Linear	20–40 Panel/Linear	10–20 Panel/Linear	Diabetic cataracts can be normal grade, soft, hard but *generally sticky*
Hold and chop	20–30 Continuous Linear	150–300 Panel/Linear	20–30 Panel/Linear	
Removal of pieces	20–30 Linear Hyperpulse/Pulse	150–250 Panel/Linear	22–28 Panel/Linear	

14. *Normal cataract with floppy iris*:

	E (%)	V (mm Hg)	FR (cc/min)	Remarks
Trench	60–70 or less Continuous Linear	20–40 Panel/Linear	10–20 Linear/Panel	
Hold and chop	20–30 Continuous Linear	200–250 Panel/Linear	24–30 Linear/Panel	
Removal of pieces	20–30 Linear Hyperpulse/Pulse	150–200 Panel/Linear	22–26 Linear/Panel	Flow rate in panel can catch iris Use of high-viscosity viscoelastic is recommended to tackle the iris

15. *Hard cataract with floppy iris*:

	E (%)	V (mm Hg)	FR (cc/min)	Remarks
Trench	60–70 Continuous Linear	20–50 Panel/Linear	10–24 Linear/Panel	Sharp tip is recommended
Hold and chop	30–40 Continuous Linear	300–350 Panel/Linear	30–34 Panel/Linear	Energy according to density of nucleus
Removal of pieces	30–35 Linear Hyperpulse/Pulse	200–300 Panel/Linear	26–32 Linear/Panel	

16. *Cataract with vitreous opacity (normal grade)*:

	E (%)	V (mm Hg)	FR (cc/min)	Remarks
Trench	60–70 Continuous Linear	20–40 Panel/Linear	10–20 Panel/Linear	
Hold and chop	20–30 Continuous Linear	250–300 Panel/Linear	20–30 Panel/Linear	
Removal of pieces	20–30 Linear Hyperpulse/Pulse	200–250 Panel/Linear	24–28 Linear/Panel	Visualization is hampered due to vitreous opacity Linear is safe

Torsional Phaco (Infinity Ozil)

- Normal cataract
- Hard cataract
- Soft cataract
- Mature cataract
- Cataract with pseudoexfoliation (normal grade)
- Cataract with hazy cornea or corneal opacity
- Very hard cataract with normal anatomy
- Cataract in post-trabeculectomized eye
- Cataract in post-vitrectomized, post-retinal detachment eye or hypotony
- Cataract with floppy iris

Phaco Parameters in Different Types of Cataract

1. *Normal cataract*:

	E (%)	V (mm Hg)	FR (cc/min)	Remarks
Trench	0–100 Linear Torsional	30–50 Panel/Linear	20–30 Panel/Linear	
Hold and chop Chop mode	30–50 Continuous Linear Longitudinal	250–350 Panel/Linear	24–34 Panel/Linear	Instead of torsional, longitudinal energy is helpful for hold
Removal of pieces Quadrant mode	0–100 Linear Torsional Intelligent Phaco (IP) on	200–300 Panel/Linear	22–32 Linear/Panel	IP is helpful Panel - procedure is fast, Linear-controlled

2. *Hard cataract*:

	E (%)	V (mm Hg)	FR (cc/min)	Remarks
Trench	0–100 Continuous Linear Torsional/ Torsional + Longitudinal (50–70)	30–50 Panel/Linear	20–30 Panel/Linear	
Hold and chop Custom I mode	30–50 Continuous Linear Longitudinal	300–400 Panel/Linear	30–40 Panel/Linear	
Removal of pieces Quadrant mode	0–100 Continuous Linear Torsional IP on	250–350 Panel/Linear	26–36 Panel/Linear	Bevel-down or bevel-up position of tip emulsifies nucleus pieces with good efficiency Use of dispersive viscoelastic to protect endothelium

3. *Soft cataract*:

	E (%)	V (mm Hg)	FR (cc/min)	Remarks
Trench	0–100 Continuous Linear Torsional	20–40 Panel/Linear	20–30 Panel/Linear	Speed of trench should be fast
Hold and chop a. Custom II mode Or	15–30 Continuous Linear Longitudinal	100–200 Panel/Linear	16–24 Linear/Panel	Custom II mode or chop mode used according to variation in density of soft cataract
b. Chop mode	15–30 Continuous Linear Longitudinal	200–250 Panel/Linear	20–30 Linear/Panel	
Removal of pieces Quadrant mode	0–100 Continuous Linear Torsional/Pulse IP on	150–200 Panel/Linear	20–30 Linear/Panel	

4. *Mature cataract*:

	E (%)	V (mm Hg)	FR (cc/min)	Remarks
Trench	0–100 Continuous Linear Torsional	30–50 Panel/Linear	20–30 Panel/Linear	Trench should be done under visualization
Hold and chop Custom I mode or chop mode	30–50 Continuous Linear Longitudinal	200–350 Panel/ Linear	24–34 Panel/ Linear	Selection of mode is according to density of nucleus
Removal of pieces Quadrant mode	0–100 Continuous Linear Torsional IP on	200–300 Panel/ Linear	20–30 Linear/ Panel	Panel can be choice for fast procedure

5. *Cataract with pseudoexfoliation (normal grade)*:

	E (%)	V (mm Hg)	FR (cc/min)	Remarks
Trench	0–100 Continuous Linear Torsional	30–50 Panel/Linear	20–30 Panel/Linear	Use of adequate energy is important to avoid pressure on zonules
Hold and chop Custom I mode or chop mode	30–50 Continuous Linear Longitudinal	200–350 Panel/Linear	24–34 Panel/Linear	
Removal of pieces Quadrant mode	0–100 Continuous Linear Torsional IP on	200–300 Panel/Linear	20–30 Linear/Panel	

6. *Cataract with hazy cornea or corneal opacity*:

	E (%)	V (mm Hg)	FR (cc/min)	Remarks
Trench	0–100 Continuous Linear Torsional	30–50 Panel/Linear	20–30 Panel/Linear	
Hold and chop Chop mode	20–30 Continuous Linear Longitudinal	250–300 Panel/Linear	24–32 Panel/Linear	
Removal of pieces Quadrant mode	0–100 Continuous Linear Torsional IP on	200–250 Panel/Linear	22–30 Linear/Panel	Bevel-down position of the tip during this step can be done due to torsional technology. Dispersive viscoelastic to protect endothelium

7. Very hard cataract with normal anatomy:

	E (%)	V (mm Hg)	FR (cc/min)	Remarks
Trench	0–100 Continuous Linear Torsional	30–50 Panel/Linear	20–30 Panel/Linear	Trench should be done slowly. Assessment of depth of groove is important
Hold and chop Custom I mode	30–60 Continuous Linear Longitudinal	250–450 Panel/Linear	30–40 Panel/Linear	Sometime (10–20%) torsional energy can be used
Removal of pieces Quadrant mode	0–100 Continuous Linear Torsional IP on	250–350 Panel/Linear	26–36 Panel/Linear	Torsional + Longitudinal (20–30%) energy can be used. Use of dispersive viscoelastic to protect endothelium

8. Cataract in post-trabeculectomized eye:

	E (%)	V (mm Hg)	FR (cc/min)	Remarks
Trench	0–100 Continuous Linear Torsional	30–50 Panel/Linear	20–30 Panel/Linear	
Hold and chop	20–30 Continuous Linear Longitudinal	250–350 Panel/Linear	26–34 Panel/Linear	According to density of nucleus
Removal of pieces Quadrant mode	0–100 Continuous Linear Torsional IP on	200–300 Panel/Linear	20–30 Linear/Panel	Uneven anterior chamber is a point of consideration in some cases

9. *Cataract in post-vitrectomized, postretinal detachment eye, or hypotony*:

	E (%)	V (mm Hg)	FR (cc/min)	Remarks
Trench	0–100 Continuous Linear Torsional	30–50 Panel/Linear	20–30 Panel/Linear	
Hold and chop Custom I mode/ chop mode	20–30 Continuous Linear Longitudinal	250–350 Panel/Linear	26–36 Panel/Linear	According to density of nucleus
Removal of pieces Quadrant mode	0–100 Continuous Linear Torsional IP on	200–300 Panel/Linear	24–34 Panel/Linear	Deep anterior chamber is the main point of concern

10. *Cataract with floppy iris*:

	E (%)	V (mm Hg)	FR (cc/min)	Remarks
Trench	0–100 Continuous Linear Torsional	30–50 Panel/Linear	20–30 Panel/Linear	
Hold and chop Chop mode	20–40 Continuous Linear Longitudinal	200–300 Panel/Linear	24–34 Panel/Linear	
Removal of pieces Quadrant mode	0–100 Continuous Linear Torsional IP on	200–250 Panel/Linear	22–32 Linear/Panel	Linear is safe to avoid catching of iris

KEY POINTS

- Setting of parameters is an important factor for successful Phaco surgery.
- Customization of these parameters varies related to different types of cataract and surgeon to surgeon (*For types of cataract, one can refer book on "Text and Atlas Slit Lamp Biomicroscopy for Assessment in Cataract Surgery"*).

CHAPTER 9

Troubleshooting

INTRODUCTION
- Troubleshooting is a very important considerable factor before, during, and after a surgical process.
- As an ophthalmologist, we are dealing with a very sensitive tissue and if the machine breaks down or fails in working, the situation is very disappointing. For this reason, one should know some important aspects of troubleshooting of Phaco machine.
- Phaco machines with their provided booklet give information related to this troubleshooting.
- During difficulties, all these machines have software, which senses the code number on the screen of console and accordingly one can refer to the booklet and check the possible causes and manage them.

DIFFICULTIES OCCURRING DURING SURGERY
Difficulties that occur during a surgery are related to the following parts and the advice is as follows:
- Phaco probe
- Tubing
- Foot pedal

Phaco Probe
1. *Phaco tip gets loosened*:

   Result:
   - Surgery is not possible
   - In a rare situation, Phaco needle may fall down in the anterior chamber.

   Advice:
   - Tighten the tip properly.

2. *Nonalignment at the junction of tip and probe*:

   Result:
   - Difficult to do surgery

Advice:
- Tip must fit in the Phaco probe socket with good alignment.

3. *Holes in the test chamber:*

    Result:
    - Leakage of the water can disturb the surgeon or the patient.

    Advice:
    - Change the test chamber.

4. *Sleeve gets torn, which is common in Kelman tip:*

    Result:
    - Heat can get transmitted to cornea.

    Advice:
    - Change the sleeve before start of surgery.

5. *Sound of occlusion without an occluded tip:*

    Result:
    - When the nuclear material is aspirated in the tip or tubing which gets blocked and hampers the Phaco fluidics, vacuum and flow rate will not work properly (especially in hard cataract).

    Advice:
    - Fill the test chamber with balanced salt solution (BSS), put the Phaco tip in the test chamber and press the foot pedal in position 3, and apply intermittent pressure on the test chamber with the fingers which helps in clearing of blocked tip, probe, or tubing.

6. *Scratches on Phaco tip or blunt Phaco tip seen under a microscope:*

    Result:
    - This can occur due to removal of very hard cataract, repeated use of tip, and by hitting of chopper with Phaco tip during hold and chop and removal of small pieces step.
    - This decreases efficiency of cutting of the nucleus.

    Advice:
    - Change the Phaco tip.

7. *Folds or scratches are noticed at the junction of Phaco probe and cable:*

    Result:
    - Acute angulation of cable attached to Phaco probe can cause kinking or damage.

CHAPTER 9

Troubleshooting

INTRODUCTION

- Troubleshooting is a very important considerable factor before, during, and after a surgical process.
- As an ophthalmologist, we are dealing with a very sensitive tissue and if the machine breaks down or fails in working, the situation is very disappointing. For this reason, one should know some important aspects of troubleshooting of Phaco machine.
- Phaco machines with their provided booklet give information related to this troubleshooting.
- During difficulties, all these machines have software, which senses the code number on the screen of console and accordingly one can refer to the booklet and check the possible causes and manage them.

DIFFICULTIES OCCURRING DURING SURGERY

Difficulties that occur during a surgery are related to the following parts and the advice is as follows:
- Phaco probe
- Tubing
- Foot pedal

Phaco Probe

1. *Phaco tip gets loosened*:

    Result:
    - Surgery is not possible
    - In a rare situation, Phaco needle may fall down in the anterior chamber.

    Advice:
    - Tighten the tip properly.

2. *Nonalignment at the junction of tip and probe*:

    Result:
    - Difficult to do surgery

Advice:
- Tip must fit in the Phaco probe socket with good alignment.

3. *Holes in the test chamber:*

   Result:
   - Leakage of the water can disturb the surgeon or the patient.

   Advice:
   - Change the test chamber.

4. *Sleeve gets torn, which is common in Kelman tip:*

   Result:
   - Heat can get transmitted to cornea.

   Advice:
   - Change the sleeve before start of surgery.

5. *Sound of occlusion without an occluded tip:*

   Result:
   - When the nuclear material is aspirated in the tip or tubing which gets blocked and hampers the Phaco fluidics, vacuum and flow rate will not work properly (especially in hard cataract).

   Advice:
   - Fill the test chamber with balanced salt solution (BSS), put the Phaco tip in the test chamber and press the foot pedal in position 3, and apply intermittent pressure on the test chamber with the fingers which helps in clearing of blocked tip, probe, or tubing.

6. *Scratches on Phaco tip or blunt Phaco tip seen under a microscope:*

   Result:
   - This can occur due to removal of very hard cataract, repeated use of tip, and by hitting of chopper with Phaco tip during hold and chop and removal of small pieces step.
   - This decreases efficiency of cutting of the nucleus.

   Advice:
   - Change the Phaco tip.

7. *Folds or scratches are noticed at the junction of Phaco probe and cable:*

   Result:
   - Acute angulation of cable attached to Phaco probe can cause kinking or damage.

Advice:
- Cable should be kept straight with respect to Phaco probe during surgery.

8. *When Phaco probe suddenly stops working (Phaco probe may be damaged):*

   Result:
   - Surgery is not possible.

   Advice:
   - Second Phaco probe should be ready or one should have a standby Phaco machine.

Tubing

1. *Tear or hole in tubing:*

   Result:
   - Spilling of water, which disturbs the surgery.
   - Water may fall down on foot pedal.

   Advice:
   - Check and change the tubing.

2. *Sometimes, damage is noticed at distal end of the tubing, which is attached to the irrigation and aspiration (I/A) line of Phaco probe:*

   Result:
   - Poor functioning of fluidics

   Advice:
   - Change the tubing.

3. *Attachment of tubing to irrigation line of Phaco probe gets loosened:*

   Result:
   - Less irrigation of fluid in the anterior chamber

   Advice:
   - Tighten the attachments.

4. *During hold and chop, vacuum did not build up:*

   Result:
   - Hold will not occur.

   Advice:
   - Problem may be in the peristaltic pump.
   - Check the rotatory movements of the pump.

5. **During quadrant removal step, suddenly Phaco fluidics does not work:**

   Result:
   - Pieces do not come toward Phaco tip or vacuum can built up without hold.
   - This is a very common situation which occurs due to clogging of nuclear pieces in the aspiration port.

   Advice:
   - Check the aspiration port of tubing and clean it.

6. *Irrigation pressure is low:*
   - Fluid in BSS bottle is less.

   Result:
   - Anterior chamber gets collapsed during surgery.
   - Surge can occur.

   Advice:
   - Replace the BSS bottle.

7. *Loose attachment of tubing to aspiration port:*

   Result:
   - Vacuum built up is less.

   Advice:
   - Check the attachments before surgery.

8. *Repeated use of tubing gives yellowish discoloration:*

   Result:
   - Functioning of Phaco fluidics is not proper

   Advice:
   - Change the tubing

9. *Air bubbles in the anterior chamber are due to excessive movement of tubing during surgery and when the assistant replaces the BSS bottle in between the surgery.*

   Result:
   - Disturbs the visualization of surgical steps

   Advice:
   - Remove all the air bubbles from the irrigation line of tubing before surgery and then start working.

10. *Sometimes, tubing will not get accepted by the machine:*

    Result:
    - Machine will not start.
    - Irrigation flow is not good from intravenous (IV) set

Advice:
- Check the irrigation flow from IV set.
- If the flow is less, change the IV set or use a wide-bore IV set.

11. *When IV set is not put properly*:

    Result:
    - Irrigation flow is less.

    Advice:
    - Join the IV set properly.

12. *Parameters are not working properly during nucleus management and I/A*:

    Result:
    - Difficulty in the step of nucleus management and irrigation aspiration

    Advice:
    - Cleaning of Phaco probe and I/A cannula should be proper after completion of case.

13. *There will be twist of tubing attached to Phaco probe or I/A cannula*:

    Result:
    - Desired direction of Phaco tip and I/A cannula will not be achieved, which disturbs the surgical step.

    Advice:
    - Attachment of these tubings in a proper direction to the Phaco probe and I/A cannula is an art.
    - It will be helpful for easy handling of Phaco probe and I/A cannula.

Foot Pedal

1. *Encircling and twisting of wire around foot pedal:*

    Result:
    - Working of foot pedal is not smooth.

    Advice:
    - Release the wire and put in proper direction.

2. *Difficulty for pressing foot pedal*:

    Result:
    - Working of foot pedal is not good.

    Advice:
    - Do the overoiling of foot pedal.
    - Do servicing of foot pedal with the machine manufacturer.

3. *Materials such as cloth, cotton balls, cotton buds, instrument, syringe, or needle can hamper the movement of foot pedal:*

   Result:
   - Working of foot pedal is not smooth.

   Advice:
   - Remove this material from foot pedal.

4. *Acute angulation of wire attached to foot pedal:*

   Result:
   - This may cause kinking or damage.

   Advice:
   - Wire should be kept at proper position.

5. *Many times, water falls down from drape with pouch on foot pedal.*

   Result:
   - Spilling of water on foot pedal can damage it.

   Advice:
   - Good quality of drape with pouch should be used.
   - It is an art of draping perfectly.

KEY POINTS

- Troubleshooting during Phaco surgery is a normal happening in a day-to-day practice.
- One can learn this troubleshooting with experience.

CHAPTER 10

Selection of Phaco Machine

INTRODUCTION

Every new practitioner is in search of a good Phaco machine:
- Selection is based on functioning of parameters of Phaco machine.
- One should have an idea about the technical and scientific aspects of the machine.
- Understanding the features and its application should correlate with each other.

PREREQUISITES

- *Performance of surgery in an ideal case of grades III and IV cataract with normal anatomy is one of the factors to select a Phaco machine.*
- One should have complete theoretical knowledge of Phaco surgery.

Selection of Phaco machine is based on the following points:
- *Diathermy:*
  - During cauterization of superficial blood vessels in limbal incision, there should not be indentation or contracture of the scleral tissue.
- *Incision:*
  - Evaluation of corneal burn at incision site is an important criteria.
- *Foot pedal:*
  - There should be perfect down and up movement of foot pedal in different positions (from I to III) in all steps of Phaco surgery.
  - *Reflux mode of foot pedal should work perfectly and is an important checkpoint.*
- *Trench:*
  - One can judge the energy performance of the machine at this step.
  - Check the irrigation flow before trench; *in other words, good irrigation flow is an important factor of consideration.*
- *Hold and chop:*
  - During hold and chop, when the vacuum and flow rate are kept in panel mode for better performance, surge should not occur.
  - *Machine which maintains the hold of nucleus for a longer duration is a very important criteria to check the efficiency of machine.*

- *Quadrant removal:*
  - Movement of pieces toward Phaco tip, i.e., Phaco fluidics is an important checkpoint.
  - If vacuum and flow rate are kept in panel/linear or at a higher side than needed in this step to check for surge
- *Irrigation and aspiration:*
  Irrigation and aspiration of epinucleus and cortex is an important step to see the efficacy of machine.
- *CAP-VAC mode:*
  According to the author, the CAP-VAC mode is an important step to check the efficacy of machine.
- *Vitrectomy:*
  - Weight of a vitrectomy cutter should be light.
  - Cutting rate should be as high as possible.
- *Important features:*
  - Machine should have different modes of energy such as continuous, burst, pulse, and hyperpulse.
  - Machine should have variable audible sounds for continuous, linear, pulse, hyperpulse mode of energy, sound of occlusion, etc.
  - Correlation of vacuum and flow rate should be in such a way that they should really assist each other in hold and chop and quadrant removal step of nucleus management.
  - Machine with minimum or no surge
  - Surgeon should feel the normal intraocular pressure in the eye during surgery.

KEY POINTS

- In this chapter, the author has mentioned points related to selection of machine in a simple way.
- Machine should be user-friendly.

Instruments Invented by Dr Navneet Toshniwal

DR TOSHNIWAL'S MICS 23G LINE OF INSTRUMENTS AND PRE CHOPPER BY SEGAL OPTIKS PVT LTD

www.segal.co.in

1. Dr Toshniwal's 23g angled titanium microcapsulorhexis forcep

Principle

Passes like needle through sideport incision and working as a forcep.

Design

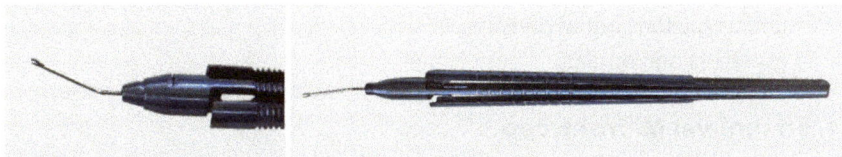

Fig. 1A

Advantages

- Due to its unique design tip, grasps the anterior capsule perfectly.
- Chances of touching to inner layers of cornea is minimal.
- Movement of this forcep inside the eye is easy.
- No pressure on anterior and posterior wall of incision site during procedure, so it maintains anterior chamber depth which is key factor for capsulorhexis.

2. Dr Toshniwal's 23g angled titanium tip microcapsule cutting scissor

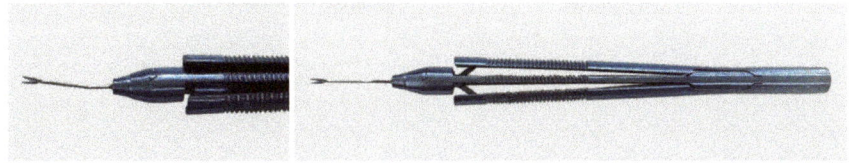

Fig. 1B

- Easy to enter through 1.2 mm incision and through sideport incision.
- Unique angle design is very convenient for the surgeon to cut the capsule.

3. Dr Toshniwal's titanium prechopper

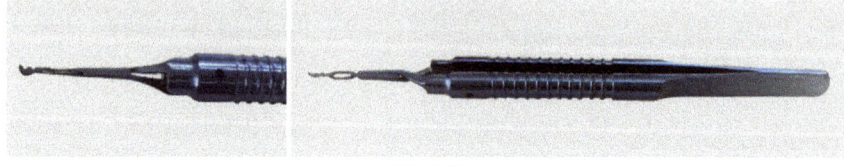

Fig. 1C

Description

- When prechopper is used in vertical fashion: Anterior surface is having two notches for better visibility of groove of trench.
- Posterior surface is curved to place the instrument parallel to posterior capsule.
- Prechopper passes throught sub2.00mm incision.

Advantages

- Nucleus division is simple and safe. Equal pressure on both halves of nucleus hastens equal division.
- Less stress on zonules.

4. Toshniwal Microforcep

Other Companies

1. Toshniwal chopper—Epsilon, UK/India (EP 107)

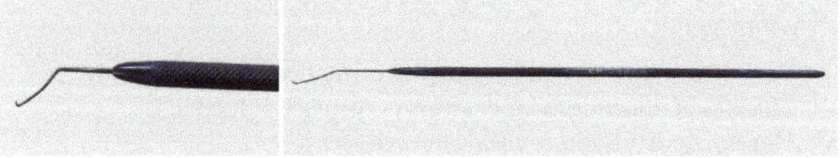

2. Toshniwal microcapsulorhexis forcep—Sunayana Surgicals, India (SST 3357)

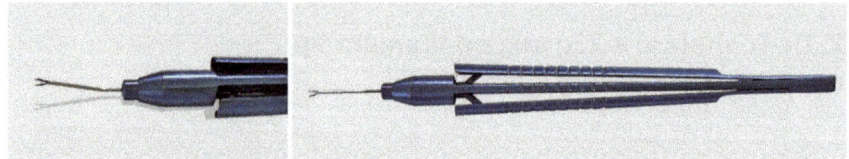

Index

Page numbers followed by *f* refer to figure and *t* refer to table.

A

Angulated tip 8, 8*f*
　　advantage of 55
Aspiration 76
　　cannula 11
Aspiration flow rate 35
　　delivery system of 37
　　hold and chop 36
　　principle 35
　　trench 36
　　uses 35

B

Burst
　　mode 16, 21
　　single 21, 22*f*

C

Cannula
　　bimanual 11
　　coaxial 11
　　types of 11
CAP-VAC mode 33, 39, 76
Cataract 57, 67
　　cortical 57, 62
　　diabetic 57, 62
　　diffuse 57, 61
　　hard 30, 32, 36, 57, 58, 63, 64
　　mature 57, 59, 65
　　normal 57-60, 64
　　　　grade of 30, 32
　　soft 29, 30, 32, 36, 57, 59, 65
　　sticky 57, 61
　　types of 56, 68
　　very hard 57, 60, 67

Cavitational effect 13
Centurion vision system 54
　　advantages 54
　　principle 54
Chop 51
Cornea
　　hazy 57
　　opacity 57, 61, 66
Cortex 52

D

Deep anterior chamber 32, 57, 59
Diathermy 12, 75
Duty cycle chart 24*t*

E

Ellips technology 26, 26*f*
　　advantages 27
　　principle 26
Energy 13
　　continuous 14, 14*f*
　　different modes of 14
　　modified modes of 23
　　principle 13
　　types of delivery system of 14
　　vacuum, and flow rate, association
　　　　of 40
　　variable whitestar 25
　　whitestar 23
Epinucleus mode 52
Eye
　　anatomy of 37
　　cataract in post-trabeculectomized
　　　　67
　　postretinal detachment 68
　　post-vitrectomized 55

Index

F

Floppy iris 57, 62, 63
    cataract with 68
Flow rate
    delivery system of 57
    different settings of 36
    parameters of 37
    principle of 35f
    role of 41
Fluid, acoustic wave of 13
Foot pedal 5, 48, 73-75
    position 6f

H

Hazy cornea, cataract with 61, 66
Hold and chop 75
Hypermetropia 57, 60
Hyperpulse energy 16, 17f
Hypotony 55

I

Ice technology 41
Incision 75
    distortion of 8f
    size of 10
Instruments 77
Intelligent phaco 43
    advantages 43
Intraocular lens 35
Intraocular pressure 55
Irrigation 76
    cannula 11
    stand 12

J

Jackhammer effect 13, 31

M

Multiburst 22, 22f
Myopia 55, 57, 59
    high 32

N

Navneet toshniwal, instruments invented by 77
Nucleus
    emulsification of 13
    management 29, 36

O

Occlusion
    effect of complete 31f
    effect of partial 31f
    mode 40, 41t
    stages 41
        postocclusion 41
        preocclusion 41
Ozil burst 49
    infinity 63
    pulse 49
Ozil continuous 49
    features of 49
    uses of 49

P

Panel mode 38
Peristaltic pump 28
Phaco
    longitudinal 13, 57
    parameters 56
    time, effective 26
    traditional 13, 57
Phaco machine 1, 56
    components of 2
    parameters of 13
    parts of 2
    selection of 75
Phaco probe 6, 69, 71, 73
    accessories 6
Phaco surgery 2, 43
    analysis of energy in 26
Phaco tip 6-9
    angulation, correlation of 7t
    anteroposterior position of 37f
    exposure of 10
    horizontal position of 37f

Index

movement of 6
types of 9
Polish 53
Pseudoexfoliation 57
    cataract with 60, 66
Pulse
    chart of long 19*t*
    chart of short 18*t*
    energy 16, 16*f*
    high-power 21, 21*f*
    long 18, 19*f*
    low-power 20, 20*f*
    per second 17*f*, 19*f*
    short 17, 17*f*
Pulse-shaping technology 42
    advantages 42
    principles 42
Pump 3
    diaphragmatic 3
    peristaltic 3, 28, 40
    venturi 3, 57
Pupil
    cataract in mid-dilated 61
    mid dilated 57
    small 29, 30, 32

Q
Quadrant removal 36, 37*f*, 51

R
Reflux 6

S
Sculpt 50
Shallow anterior chamber 29, 32, 60
Silicon material, high-quality 10
Sleeve, thickness of 10
Span, general position for 48*f*
Straight tip 7*f*
Stroke length 14
Surge 43
    avoid 45
    complications to 44
    factors responsible for 44
    mechanism of 44*f*
Surgery, difficulties occurring during 69

T
Titanium microcapsulorhexis forcep 77
Titanium tip microcapsule cutting scissor 77
Torsional amplitude 47
Torsional phaco 63
Torsional technology 46, 46*f*
    advantages 46
    disadvantages 54
    machine features 47
    principle 46
    surgical parameters 50
Toshniwal chopper 78
Toshniwal microcapsulorhexis forcep 78
Toshniwal microforcep 78
Toshniwal titanium prechopper 78
Trans-urethral resection 45
Trench 15*f*, 75
Tubing 71
    repeated use of 72
    set 4

V
Vacuum 28
    adequate 34
    delivery system of 33, 57
    different settings of 29
    linear mode 33
    panel mode 34
    principle 28
    role of 31
    use of 28, 31
Viscoelastic removal 53
Viscoelastic solution, removal of 33, 39
Vitrectomy 76
    anterior 54
    cutter 12
Vitreous opacity 57
    cataract with 63

W
Wound, distortion of 9*f*

Z
Zonules 32
    weak 55

EU GSPR Authorised Reprsentative
Logos Europe, 9 rue Nicolas Poussin
1700, La Rochelle, France
Phone: +33 (0) 6 67 93 73 78
E-mail: contact@logoseurope.eu